"The feminine as transgression and as the 'other' by excellence, these are some of the ideas put forward in this book, which offers a deep exploration of the masculine and feminine, the difference, which is paradigmatic of all other differences, in the words of Francoise Heritier. The author is innovative, challenging and inspiring. The book is a must read for all those interested in this topic."

—**Rosine Perelberg**, *Distinguished Fellow, British Psychoanalytic Society; Sigourney Prize winner 2023; author,* Sexualité, Excès et Représentation

"Jacqueline Schaeffer knows very well adolescents and the intensity of the conflicts they face. She captures the essence of the complex issue of the refusal of the feminine in our society, and of the stimulating work of psychoanalytic technique with contemporary patients. She restores the body issues to central position and offers rich and radical reflections on working with young patients facing conflicts towards bisexuality that leads to the repudiation of the feminine. This is a brilliant book, exciting and very accessible: a good combination of education and psychoanalytic thinking."

—**Christine Anzieu-Premmereur**, *MD, PhD, Assistant Clinical Professor in Psychiatry at Columbia University; Chair IPA COCAP, Co-Founder, Pulsion Psychoanalytic Institute, New York*

"This crucial book deals with the themes of otherness, what it means to 'be a woman' or 'to have the sense of being a woman', and of 'being recognized as a woman'. Jacqueline Schaeffer explores their multiple facets: how girls become aware of their femininity, the censorship of the woman-as-lover, the conflict between the feminine and maternal spheres, the difference between the sexes as a paradigm of all differences, and so on. Finally, she considers the derailments or failures of the feminine sphere as taboos. All of this makes fascinating reading."

—**Marilia Aisenstein**, *Psychoanalyst, Paris Psychoanalytical Society (SPP) and British Association of Psychoanalysis (BRAS)*

Psychoanalysis and the Feminine

Psychoanalysis and the Feminine presents Jacqueline Schaeffer's understanding of the feminine as a psychoanalytic concept.

Schaeffer considers the difference between the sexes to be the paradigm of all differences, and the basis for the repudiation of the feminine and gender theories, those that destitute or invalidate psychic bisexuality. In addition, the author proposes a number of oppositions: a feminine, constructed in relation to the masculine, which differentiates itself from the person of the woman, and also from femininity; a feminine that distinguishes itself from the phallic, which denies its existence, hates it or wants to dominate it; a feminine that is antagonistic to but not cleaved from the maternal, with which it can be harmoniously reconciled; a feminine that carries the risk of suffering, but also the chance of a destiny of openness and growth.

Psychoanalysis and the Feminine: An Other Sex will be key reading for psychoanalysts in practice and in training, and for students of psychoanalytic studies, gender studies and feminist philosophy.

Jacqueline Schaeffer is an honorary training and supervising analyst of the Psychoanalytical Society of Paris, France. She is former editor of the *Revue Française de Psychanalyse* and the *Débats de psychanalyse*, and a former supervisor in child and adolescent psychotherapy at the Pierre Male Child Guidance Center, Sainte Anne Hospital in Paris.

Routledge Focus on Mental Health

Routledge Focus on Mental Health presents short books on current topics, linking in with cutting-edge research and practice.

Titles in the series:

Understanding and Coping with Illness Anxiety
Phil Lane

The Linguistic Turn of the English Renaissance: A Lacanian Perspective
Shirley Zisser

The Concept of the Individual in Psychoanalysis: The Ego, the Self, the Subject, and the Person
Raul Moncayo

A Critical Reconstruction of Evidence-based Practice in Psychology: Evidence and Ethics
Henrik Berg

Physician Wellness and Resilience: Narrative Prompts to Address Burnout
Pauline Davies and Cynthia M. Stonnington

Psychoanalysis and the Feminine: An "Other" Sex
Jacqueline Schaeffer
Translated by Andrew Weller

For a full list of titles in this series, please visit https://www.routledge.com/Routledge-Focus-on-Mental-Health/book-series/RFMH

Psychoanalysis and the Feminine

An "Other" Sex

Jacqueline Schaeffer

Translated by Andrew Weller

Routledge
Taylor & Francis Group
LONDON AND NEW YORK

First published in English 2025
by Routledge
4 Park Square, Milton Park, Abingdon, Oxon OX14 4RN

and by Routledge
605 Third Avenue, New York, NY 10158

Routledge is an imprint of the Taylor & Francis Group, an informa business

First Published in French as Le Féminin: un sexe autre de Jacqueline Schaeffer. © 2022 by IN PRESS ÉDITIONS.

British Library Cataloguing-in-Publication Data
A catalogue record for this book is available from the British Library

ISBN: 9781032748184 (hbk)
ISBN: 9781032748153 (NIP) (pbk)
ISBN: 9781003471042 (ebk)

DOI: 10.4324/9781003471042

Typeset in Times New Roman
by codeMantra

For Justine

Contents

About the Author

Jacqueline Schaeffer is an honorary full member and training analyst of the Paris Psychoanalytical Society. In 1986, she was awarded the Maurice Bouvet prize in psychoanalysis. She is a former editor of the *Revue française de Psychanalyse* and a former assistant editor of the "Psychoanalytic debates" series with the Presses Universitaires de France. She has published several papers and been the keynote speaker in many conferences throughout the world. Her book, *The Universal Refusal: A Psychoanalytic Exploration of the Feminine Sphere and its Repudiation* was published by Karnac Books in 2011.

Introduction

An "other" rather than "second" feminine sex

In what follows I am taking the bold step of using the noun "feminine," while at the same time being very careful to differentiate it from the world of women, for everyone knows that each woman is unique. And, further, I argue that the feminine can only be defined in terms of transgression. My choice is to consider the feminine sex as "other" rather than "second" (de Beauvoir, 1953/1949).

Freud (1918) puts it unequivocally:

> Perhaps this dread is based on the fact that woman is different from man, forever incomprehensible and mysterious, strange and therefore apparently hostile. The man is afraid of being weakened by the woman, infected with her femininity and of then showing himself incapable.
>
> (pp. 198–199)

Is the expression of this dread a characteristic of Freud himself or is it solely attributed to primitive man? *Non liquet*. At any rate, it is well known that there is a primitive man nestling within every civilized being. A woman may therefore be perceived as "other," hostile and castrating.

Could it not be said that a feeling of disquieting and familiar strangeness is the prerogative of the feminine dimension of a woman? How can we fail to link this "other" to what Freud (1915) describes as primal hate: "At the very beginning, it seems, the external world, objects and what is hated are identical" (p. 136). A few lines above he writes: "The ego has separated off a part of its own self, which it projects into the external world and feels as hostile" (ibid).

This is what gave rise to the famous dictum: "the object emerges in hate." Freud considers that it is a primary defence at the level of self-preservation, before being applied to the register of sexuality.

What Freud refers to as "a part of this great riddle of sex," namely, "the repudiation of femininity" (in my terms, the refusal to acknowledge the feminine sphere) thus becomes a little less enigmatic. It is a protective measure.

But what about the maternal sphere, then, since the first woman of all human beings is the mother? I shall be careful to differentiate between the feminine sphere and the maternal sphere.

"One is not born, but rather becomes a woman," Simone de Beauvoir (1953/1949, p. 301) wrote. One is not born a woman, of course! But one is born a baby of female sex. From being girls we become women, and often mothers. But the erotic and libidinal feminine sphere, in the sense that it is important to differentiate it from femininity, is something that has to be conquered, something that has to be wrested.

"My body is mine!" it was proclaimed in 1968. But, alas, no! The female body is also, first and foremost, an object to be conquered, to be freed from the body, attraction and ascendancy of the primitive mother. It is dependent on the forces of destiny in the form of periods – the first time, and then every month thereafter – pregnancy, childbirth and the menopause.

It must also try to wrest itself from the force of internal objects which, when they become fixed as *imagos*, are tyrants that prevent some human beings from living, loving and experiencing moments of happiness, but above all from creating their own history and becoming the full subjects of their lives. Psychoanalysis, thanks to transference, offers them a solution, a chance to take control of their own inner freedom, that is to say, the possibility of feeling neither victim nor guilty, but responsible for their own drives.

All the stages in a woman's life are experiences, very often trials, that require large amounts of energy and, as Freud (1915) says of the pressure of the drives, a "demand for work" (p. 122).

The most decisive stage in psychosexual development is that of the Oedipal organization, linked to the cathexis of the difference between the sexes and to identifications with the parents or progenitors of both sexes. It is underpinned by a sexual identity based on biological certainty and confirmed by the parental environment.

But the trajectory of this oedipal organization is extended and completed by a decisive experience, based on an encounter: that of a sexual relationship of ecstatic pleasure (*jouissance*) which finally reveals to a woman the erotic essence of her sexual organs, and therefore of her feminine sphere.

I am therefore offering a psychoanalytical conception of the feminine sphere insofar as it is formed in relation to the masculine sphere, differentiated from the person of the woman and from femininity, and antagonistic to, yet not split off from, the maternal sphere, while bringing with it the risks of suffering but also opportunities for a destiny of openness and fulfilment.

References

Beauvoir, S. de. (1953/1949). *The Second Sex*, trans. and edited by Parshley, H.M., with an introduction by Crosland, M. New York: Alfred A. Knopf, 1993.

Freud, S. (1915). Instincts and their vicissitudes. *S. E., 14*. London: Hogarth, pp. 117–140.

Freud, S. (1918 [1917]). The taboo of virginity (contributions to the psychology of love, III). *S. E., 11*. London: Hogarth, pp. 193–208.

Chapter 1

The other and the object

The four figures of the other

At the very beginning of mental life, Freud (1915) tells us, the external world is not libidinally cathected. It is "indifferent" (p. 136).

He goes on to describe primal hatred, which is said to be a first necessary operation of differentiation, a primal splitting. He writes: "At the very beginning, the outside world, the object and what is hated are identical" (p. 136). For Freud, the other and the object do not seem to be differentiated.

The first "other" is the *Nebenmensch*, the fellow human being, who is challenged by the infant's state of distress and need for care. It is a prefiguration of the object.

But, for Freud, it is when the object makes its appearance during the stage of primary narcissism that the variable of pleasure/unpleasure, then that of love/hate, come into play. He writes:

> For the pleasure-ego, the external world is divided into a part that is pleasurable, which it has incorporated into itself, and a remainder that is extraneous to it. It has separated off a part of its own self, which it projects into the external world and feels as hostile.
>
> (Freud, 1915, p. 136)

This is what gave rise to the famous statement that "the object emerges in hate." Freud considers that this is a first defence of the ego even before it is applied to the register of sexuality: "The hate which is admixed with the love is in part derived from the preliminary stages of loving; it is also in part based on reactions of repudiation by the ego-instincts" (Freud, 1915, p. 139). It is the root, Freud was to say, of misogyny, racism and anti-Semitism.

If the other is to constitute itself as an object, it must therefore leave the field of non-cathexis, indifference or unpleasure for a cathexis in love/hate.

Conversely, would an object attacked by decathexis, destructiveness or de-objectalization be excorporated from the ego? Would it then become again an indifferent "other"? Or would it remain contaminated by hate? In which

DOI: 10.4324/9781003471042-1

case, its objectality would only be amplified, since hate is older and stronger than love, and strongly maintains its object.

André Green (1996) asks, "Does sexuality have anything to do with psychoanalysis?" (p. 831). It is a surprising question. How could they really be dissociated?

Freud made infantile sexuality and sexual development his launching pad. Sexuality is at the origins of human life and is sexually transmissible. The desire for a child (which is hard to imagine being asexual) and the difference between the sexes haunt maternal reverie. At birth, the first look and the first words raise the question: Is it a boy or girl?

In connection with sexuality and the difference between the sexes, the process of otherness encounters a series of "figures of the other," whose emergence generates shock effects. These shocks, which will later be called "crises," are an opportunity for the mind because they force it to reorganize its perception of the world and to reshape instinctual drive functioning.

Here is a brief description, which will be described in more detail in the following chapters. The first stages of life presuppose a state of non-differentiation, a fusional dyad, formulated by Freud (1941) as follows: "The breast is a part of me, I am the breast" (p. 299). A primary identification and a first cathexis of cannibalistic, oral incorporation are indistinguishable, which concern both the child and the mother who has sheltered and fantasized about the child in her womb.

Maternal care and the mother's mirror gaze are present. The mother, the first seductress, awakens the child's erogenous zones.

The first figure of the other

This occurs when the mother returns to her sexual night in the marital bed. It is a first antagonism between the feminine and the maternal spheres.

The mother then carries out what has been theorized in terms of the "censorship of the woman as lover" (*censure de l'amante*) (Braunschweig & Fain, 1975): a transmission, through her own body, of a mediated message designating an "other" of her desire. For the child, a very first process of otherness emerges. The child's vision of the world is turned upside down. The mother becomes "an other"; she is no longer "me." But what's more, there is an "other of the other." So we move from one to three.

It is not yet an object, but a proto-cathexis, a precursor of the creation of an object. Could it be an "object cathected before it is perceived," as Serge Lebovici (1960) theorized? Or rather a proto-object, cathected while it is still perceived as a part of oneself (narcissistic-related object), before it is truly perceived as external to oneself (object-related object). This seems to relate to Winnicott's (1971a) distinction between subjective objects and objective objects.

The child's first mental operations when faced with this initial shock are the hallucination of satisfaction and the first manifestations of autoeroticism.

This is certainly a decisive moment in the first colouring of excitation by the drives. "On its path from its source to its aim," writes Freud (1933), "the instinct becomes psychically operative" (p. 96).

The "mental" register does not exist in itself; it is what becomes active in the drive circuit.

This drive circuit involves a double "reversal," that is to say, reversal into its opposite and turning round upon the subject's own self. According to Freud, this is a "first attempt by the ego to defend itself" against instinctual demands before repression occurs, "which cannot arise until a sharp cleavage has occurred between conscious and unconscious mental activity" (Freud, 1915, p. 147).

As André Green (1999/1993) emphasizes, it is the very prototype of a negativity that is accomplished under the effect of the sole thrust of the unconscious and prior to repression, as the basic defences of the nascent mental apparatus. Could objectalization, then, be the product of a "work of the negative"?

The second figure of the other

This is an anatomical perception: the sight of a penis, or the absence of one. Rather than a difference, it is more of an all-or-nothing division. The view of the world is once again turned upside down. "Throne and Altar are in danger," writes Freud (1927, p. 153).

This shock gives rise to a very powerful mental operation of "primal repression" which projects all the content of this experience, despite its intensity, into the unconscious of the infantile amnesia. It is almost impossible to recover memories before the age of four. The shock is repressed, but it will have retroactive effects.

How does the transition from otherness to the construction of the object occur? On the side of the drives, it is infantile sexuality, spurred on by curiosity, that leads to the libidinal development of a child and the eroticization of its erogenous zones. This evolution contributes to the construction of the child's ego and to the child's liberation from the primitive mother. On the side of thought, a child invents infantile sexual theories that are an attempt to answer the great riddles of humanity, namely, conception, birth, sexuality and death.

Another powerful mental operation is produced by this shock: "denial." This denial is involved in the creation of an infantile sexual theory, the theory of phallic monism. This phallic organization attributes excessive narcissistic value to a single sex, the penis, erected as a phallus, and gives its bearer an assurance of power and a value of superiority, which will tend to persist in the form of male domination. At the same time, the identificatory solution takes into account the difference between the sexes, that of the progenitors or parents.

The operation of the "double reversal" is essential here. The most important one is the turning round upon the subject's own self, and what Freud called the "reflexive middle voice" (1915, p. 128), which gives access to reflexivity and internalization.

But this operation also plays a part in the process of objectalization when, in the double reversal described by Freud, the participation of an object is involved: "An extraneous person is once more sought as an object; this person, in consequence of the alteration which has taken place in the instinctual aim, has to take over the role of the subject" (Freud, 1915, p. 127).

This refers both to the "use of the object," according to Winnicott (1971b) but also to the notion of "subject" and that of "subjectivation," each of which will have their moment of glory.

The third figure of the other

This is the female sexual organ. The great discovery, at puberty, is the appearance of a new female organ: the vagina. The view of the world is once again turned upside down. The difference between the sexes can no longer be denied. The castration complex no longer has the same configuration or the same function.

The fourth figure of the other

This fourth figure is that of the loving and sexual encounter. The shock of the feminine sphere may or may not be worked through and integrated with the advent of the first sexual relations, in both sexes.

The other has become an object, but one that maintains its characteristic of otherness. "Perhaps this dread is based on the fact," writes Freud (1918), "that woman is different from man, forever incomprehensible and mysterious, strange and therefore apparently hostile. The man is afraid of being weakened by the woman, infected with her femininity and of then showing himself incapable" (pp. 198–199).

The double reversal initiates the processes of identification necessary for working through and integrating psychic bisexuality. The transformation of the "other" into an object may fail if an affect of terror or disgust arises. For a man, a woman may not be constituted as a whole object and remain a "part-object," of a fetishistic nature. The other object, whether one is a man or a woman, is always the feminine component.

References

Braunschweig, D., & Fain, M. (1975). *La nuit, le jour. Essai psychanalytique sur le fonctionnement mental.* Paris: Presses Universitaires de France.

Freud, S. (1915). Instincts and their vicissitudes. *S.E.* 14. London: Hogarth, pp. 117–140.

Freud, S. (1918 [1917]). The taboo of virginity. *S.E.* 11. London: Hogarth, pp. 193–208.

Freud, S. (1927). Fetishism. *S.E.* 21. London: Hogarth, pp. 152–157.

Freud, S. (1933). New Introductory Lectures to Psychoanalysis. *S.E. 22*. London: Hogarth, pp. 1–182.

Freud, S. (1941 [1938]). Findings, ideas, problems. *S.E.* 23. London: Hogarth, pp. 299–300.

Green, A. (1996). La sexualité a-t-elle un quelconque rapport avec la psychanalyse? *Revue française de psychanalyse*, 60(3): 829–847.

Green, A. (1999/1993). *The Work of the Negative*, trans. Andrew Weller. London: Free Association Books.

Lebovici, S. (1960). La relation objectale chez l'enfant. *Psychiatrie de l'enfant*, 3(1): 147–226.

Winnicott, D. (1971a). The split off male and female elements to be found clinically in men and women. In: *Playing and Reality.* London: Tavistock, pp. 72–85.

Winnicott, D. (1971b). The use of an object and relating through identifications. In: *Playing and Reality.* London: Tavistock, pp. 86–94.

Chapter 2

The difference between the sexes

The paradigm of all differences

> "There is one particularly constant relation between femininity and instinctual life"
>
> Freud (1933, p. 116)

Is it a girl or boy? This is the first question when a child is born. It is through sexuality and the difference between the sexes that the child comes into the world. It is the first difference, paradigmatic of all differences (Héritier, 1966).

The first difference is the other, and the other, from the very beginning, is the other sex. Unless the sex is first established via an ultrasound scan, the sight of the sexual organs precedes the naming of gender. The name of the sex presides over all identity.

This anatomy is inaugurated like a destiny. But nothing could be less certain when it comes to human nature, which is not governed by sexuality and instinct but nourished by history, fantasies and tyrannized by imagos and conflicts. It is a hijacked, "denatured" sexuality (André, 2019), and thus a psychosexuality.

The riddle that has forever puzzled psychoanalysts and ordinary people alike is that of the difference between the sexes. If extraterrestrials were to honour us with a visit of the third kind, their most startling surprise, Freud suggested, would be this discovery.

This difference is as banal as it is irreducible. But it is a difference that imposes such a demand upon the mind for work that every individual, child or adult, man or woman, philosopher or scientist, whether in a couple or in society, strives to deploy all the tricks of a counterforce of equal magnitude to attenuate or erase its effects.

As Freud wrote to Ernest Jones on 17 May 1914: "Anyone who promises to mankind liberation from the hardship of sex will be welcomed as a hero, let him talk whatever nonsense he chooses" (Pauskaskas, 1993, p. 297). In fact, what does violence to the ego, at every age, is the intrapsychic conflict of the difference between the sexes.

DOI: 10.4324/9781003471042-2

Psychosexual identity

The human infant must face the shock of the anatomical discovery of the difference between the sexes. It must then build its psychosexual identity mentally. This identity is the result of libidinal development linked to the cathexis of the difference between the sexes and identifications with the parents or progenitors of both sexes. It first requires a sexual identity, based on the biological certainty of belonging to a specific anatomical sex, which is confirmed by the parents.

"Whatever our sexuality may be," writes Michel Schneider (2007),

> it is related to the difference between the sexes, even and especially when it aims to transgress this difference. There is no such thing as asexuation or asexuality. We are not human without being a man or a woman. We are not human before being a man or a woman
>
> (p. 127)

I argue that psychosexual identity, on the path that leads to the masculine/feminine pairing, is not acquired definitively, because it has to be constructed and maintained permanently due to the constancy of the libidinal pressure and the conflict of the difference between the sexes. It also has to be modulated in relation to psychic bisexuality which also plays a role in it.

This is why it is essential not to confuse sexual identity with the choice of sexual object, nor identity with identification, nor sexual identity with gender identity.

- The term *identity* refers to the questions: "Who is he? Who am I?", "What sex is he?" "What sex am I?"
- *Identification* describes an unconscious process of integrating the other, or an aspect of the other, into oneself, which insensitively transforms the subject: the question asked is: "Who has come into me? Who inhabits me?"
- *Gender identity* corresponds to a current trend that originated in the United States and has spread throughout the whole of Europe. It consists in neglecting the biological sex, seen as a secondary variable, in favour of a construction, self-determination, a choice of gender, one gender among many genders (see below).

I argue that it is the "work of the feminine sphere," for both men and women, that ensures access to the difference between the sexes and the preservation, albeit conflictual, of psychosexual identity. I shall come back to this later. This identity remains unstable, however, because it requires constant work and is constantly threatened by regression to the active/passive opposition or to the phallic/castrated pairing, both of which relieve the ego of the "demand for work" made upon it in the face of the constant pressure of the sexual drives.

If, as Simone de Beauvoir says, "One is not born a woman, one becomes one," I would say that the feminine sphere, like the masculine sphere, at the genital level, is not something acquired at puberty, as Freud suggests, with the experience of the first sexual relations, but is a conquest that has to be constantly renewed, spurred on by the constant libidinal pressure.

Femininity and drive life

Freud moved away from nature, the nature of instinct, but without ever setting biology aside, to explore a new territory, that of drive activity and "psychization," in other words, rendering excitation psychically operative.

According to the Freudian drive theory to which I am referring, the libido imposes a conflict on the ego which must organize various means of defence. It postulates a pathway from unavoidable internal excitation which, from its bodily source to its aim of seeking satisfaction, becomes psychically operative by attaining the status of a drive (Freud, 1933, p. 96). If excitation does not manage to become psychically operative as a drive, or if the drive degrades into excitation, there is an emergence of so-called "psychosomatic" disorders, addiction-related pathologies, acting-out and so on.

The sexual drive, the libido, has an essential predicate called "constant force." This pressure is a fundamental anthropological transformation of evolution starting from the periodic thrusts of instinct.

As Freud (1915) insisted, an instinct "never operates as a momentary force giving a *momentary* impact, but always as a *constant* one" (p. 118). And in 1933, after the turning point of 1920 and the advent of the last drive theory, he wrote: "On its path from its source to its aim, the instinct becomes operative psychically." And again: "A constant force… that the subject cannot avoid by flight… It is from this pressing that it derives its name of *Trieb*" (Freud, 1933, p. 96). Jacques Lacan (1963) agrees:

> The constancy of the thrust forbids any assimilation of the drive to a biological function, which always has a rhythm... It has no day or night, no spring or autumn, no rise and fall. It is a constant force...
>
> (p. 165)

Indeed, this constant thrust ignores the seasons, those of childhood and ageing. Its strength may vary, but its constancy remains unchanging. Can we not infer from this that the "drive impulse," which defines the "id" of the second topography, also inherits this "constant thrust"?

This constant thrust does violence to the ego, which has to adapt to rhythm and time, and, as Freud writes, it imposes on it a "demand for work." It is in this way that the ego is differentiated from the "id," that excitation becomes drive, that human genitality is differentiated from animal sexuality, subject to rutting periods and the *oestrus*. Human sexuality is a psychosexuality, and human desire is driven by psychical life. It goes without saying that I am taking into account here the relational context in which this libidinal force exerts itself and the response to it.

But in 1912, Freud considered that, unlike need, which can be satisfied by appropriate action, "something in the nature of the sexual instinct itself is unfavourable to the realization of complete satisfaction!" (Freud, 1912, p. 188). If the drive were to be satisfied, why would it continue to press, and what would become of desire?

It was the difficulty of theorizing the feminine sexual component in terms of the inevitable constant pressure of large libidinal quantities that induced Freud to put forward the notion of an insurmountable "repudiation of femininity" (or, as I put it, of the refusal to acknowledge the feminine sphere), in the form of penis envy or the repudiation of homosexual passivity. I shall come back to this.

The psychosexual pairings according to Freud

Let me recall briefly that Freud describes the development of psychosexuality, which is essential at the level of the construction of the ego for its cathexes and its defences, in terms of three pairings.

A first *active/passive* pairing, the so-called "anal" organization, concerns the acquisition of sphincter control and motricity. The ego acquires its sovereignty from this organization of activity/passivity and control. This is the moment that can be identified, through observation, when a young child says "no" and "I am all alone." The "ego/I" manifests itself, it can say yes or no to its drive and also to the object. This is the moment when it can make the main differentiations between the ego and not-ego, inside and outside, good and bad, clean and dirty, etc. It is a platform, a marshalling yard, and a first possibility for the subject to free him or herself from the maternal object.

The moment of the sensory pleasures of orality is only a prelude to the constitution of the ego. The oral impulse is above all carnal, bodily, a prelude to the intrapsychic dimension and the constitution of the ego, which is not yet altogether distinct from the maternal primary object. It is not possible as yet to speak of an intrapsychic pairing. The oral impulse is the crucible of the experience of ecstatic pleasure, so much so that Freud considers the infant satisfied at the breast to be the prototype of the sexual relation of ecstatic pleasure.

Freud then describes a second pairing: that of the *universal penis/neutered penis*, during the stage of "phallic" organization, when the shock of the discovery of the difference between the sexes occurs, which consists in recognizing only one sex, the penis. This pairing leads to the construction of the Oedipus complex, an essential organizer of psychosexuality and identifications with two objects of different sex.

Finally, Freud discusses the *male/female* pairing, which for him only exists at puberty, at the so-called "genital" stage, at the moment of encounter and the possible achievement of the sexual act.

I want to emphasize the fact that while the active/passive pairing designates a pair of opposites or polarities, and the *phallic/castrated* pairing a mode of functioning in terms of all or nothing, only the *male/female pairing* designates a real difference, the difference between the sexes.

The discovery of the difference between the sexes

Freud describes the perceptual ordeal of the discovery of the difference between the sexes as a trauma that mobilizes, in both boys and girls, intense cathectic and anti-cathectic energy. "Throne and Altar are in danger," he says, where power and religion are recognized.

This ordeal is worked through, in a structuring way, through the Oedipal conflict, by means of two solutions: a phallic solution and an identificatory solution.

The first, the phallic solution, is to deny the difference between the sexes, driven by castration anxiety, which consists in recognizing only one sexual organ, the penis, the only visible one, and differentiating humans into those who have one and those who do not.

The second, the identificatory solution, takes into account the difference between the sexes as well as the difference between parents or progenitors, and leads to the renunciation of incestuous wishes, the internalization of the superego, and the onset of latency.

Sexuality and femininity

In 1905, in publishing his *Three Essays on the Theory of Sexuality*, Freud created two scandals: infantile sexuality and perversely predisposed adult sexuality. This respectable 49-year-old man was deemed malignant and obscene, and people stopped greeting him in the street.

Under the veil of a riddle, he left a third scandal, a "dark continent" to be explored: that of female sexuality, or rather the sexuality of women. Freud had nonetheless had the opportunity to explore this dark continent. At the Salpêtrière hospital he had come into contact with many women said to be "hysterical," and it was one of them in particular who enabled him to invent the psychoanalytical situation, the woman who said to him in so many words, "Don't touch me, listen to me!"

It was then that Freud was able to develop his theory of the drives, once he had decided to abandon what he called his "*neurotica,*" the causality of an event, and turn to the psychic world of fantasy, in particular the fantasy of seduction.

We know that his writings on the difference between the sexes and the Oedipus complex came much later, in the 1920s, and that his writings on femininity appeared in the 1930s, after the death of his mother. But how many feminine notations there are in writings such as "Dora," "The taboo of virginity," and in all his literary texts, which have the potential for shedding light on this obscure continent!

Which feminine sphere?

I do not accept a definition in terms of "gender" either for the feminine sphere or the masculine sphere. Gender is not a psychoanalytical notion, since the purpose of analysis is not to accept it as such but to question it in terms of narcissistic and object-related cathexis, or in terms of identifications. I have chosen to reserve the term "feminine" for the time of the test of otherness and the conceptual meaning of one of the terms of a difference: the difference between the sexes.

In Chapter 3, "Preludes to the feminine sphere," I will look at theorizations designating a "primal feminine sphere" of sexuality (André, 1995), a "primary feminine sphere" (Guignard, 1997), or a "pure feminine element" (Winnicott, 1971). All of these refer to a "primeval era," which is not situated at the level of the advent of the male/female difference of the sexes for the subject, but at the time of the impregnations and first identifications with the maternal feminine sphere or the mother's sexuality, and therefore with a primary maternal dimension.

Moreover, I differentiate between the feminine sphere, the sphere of the flesh, the interior and the invisible, carrying all the fantasies of danger, and femininity, which is visible, the sphere of the body, seduction, deception and masquerade, which goes well with the phallic dimension and reassures castration anxiety, in both men and women.

The bedrock of the repudiation of the feminine sphere

Having established the difference between the male and female sexes at the moment of puberty, Freud theoretically called it into question, and a fourth pairing emerged: *bisexuality and the repudiation of the feminine sphere* in both sexes.

It was in the twilight of his life, in 1937, after having set the Charybdis of the death drive in 1920 against the drives of life and love, that Freud designated the Scylla of the "repudiation of femininity" (or, in my terms, of the feminine sphere) in both sexes, the bedrock on which therapeutic efforts break down. He referred to it as "a part of the great riddle of sexuality."

Faced with the difficulties and failures encountered in his analytical work, was this not a way for him of reintroducing the sexual drive, of restoring to it the demonic capacity that he had taken away from it and of giving it back the same disruptive polarity that he had attributed to the death drive?

It is interesting to note that the formulations Freud uses show the extent to which what he designates as "genital" is difficult to separate from the pre-genital precursors, anal and phallic, and the so-called "part" objects. Thus, Freud (1917), took up Lou Andréas Salomé's expression according to which the vagina was "taken on lease from the rectum" (p. 133). The penis can be likened to a "faecal stick." The female sex organ is defined in relation to the penis, as an appendage: "the vagina is now valued as a place of shelter for the penis" (Freud, 1923, p. 145). And when Freud talks about penis envy and its vicissitudes, he uses the expression "man as an appendage of the penis"!

With the term "bedrock," Freud induces a pessimistic point of view about sexuality, which designates, without explicitly saying so, both sexual impotence and the analyst's powerlessness to remedy it.

In Freud's view, women remain riveted to their desire for the penis – which is partly true – and men to their homosexual dread of being penetrated. In my view, in both cases they are pregenital defences against anxiety to do with genital penetration, anxiety about a vagina that has to let itself be penetrated or that has to be penetrated by a libidinal penis. It is therefore much more to do with the difference between the sexes, at the level of the sexual relation itself.

Furthermore, it is remarkable that it is the feminine sphere, the eternal disrupter of the social order and the process of civilization, that is designated, here once again, in the sexual domain, as threatening psychosexual identity and endangering the unstable alloy of the psychic bisexual nucleus common to both sexes.

The "bedrock of the repudiation of the feminine sphere" is active in all of us, and the fantasies and ideas attached to it raise a defensive shield, both theoretical and clinical. No individual, man or woman, is willing to expose themselves to a personal questioning of their prejudices, sexual practices or sexual theories that are still active. "The psychoanalyst must remain the erogenous zone of society," said the psychoanalyst Michel Fain.

Neurosis and sexuality are no longer at the forefront of the reflections of psychoanalysts today. A number of preoccupying issues may justify this. But how can we accept that actual adult sexuality is so rarely part of their field of theoretical exploration? Can we not infer from this forms of resistance akin to the rock of the "repudiation of the feminine sphere" that lies dormant in all of us? But why the feminine sphere?

It is interesting to note that both the new pairing of bisexuality and the rejection of the feminine component in both sexes, and each of the terms in this pairing, taken separately, point to a negation of the difference between the sexes.

- On the one hand, the repudiation of the feminine sphere is a refusal to acknowledge what, in the difference between the sexes, is most alien and most difficult to include within an anal or phallic logic, namely the female genitals. The female genitals are invisible, secret, unfamiliar and the source of all kinds of dangerous fantasies. They are disturbing for men because they reflect an image, a representation, of castrated sexual organs that makes them fear for their own genitals. But, above all, it is because the openness of the female body, its quest for sexual ecstatic pleasure and its ability to admit large quantities of constant libidinal thrust is a source of anxiety for both men and women.

- On the other hand, psychic bisexuality can also represent a negation of the difference between the sexes, as will be explained below.

It would therefore seem that accession to the distinction between the sexes does not constitute a platform of stability and security, and that it is legitimate to claim that what Freud refers to as a bedrock is that of the difference between the sexes.

Infantile sexual theories

It is the perception of the difference between the sexes that drives the child, as we know, to engage in an intense activity of thought, to the point of developing infantile sexual theories. The enigma of the other and infantile sexuality are constitutive of the unconscious.

The infantile sexual theories noted by Freud are constructs that provide answers to essential questions: where do children come from, how are they made, what happens between parents, what is death? Constructed in terms of a child's libidinal development, they turn children into young scientists and philosophers before they enter the Oedipal situation, as they question the great enigmas of humanity: conception, birth, sexuality and death.

Adults feel the need to invent theoretical systems and technical solutions to these enigmas, using science, religion, philosophy and other means, including the most aberrant ones: those of the mad scientist, the mad philosopher, the religious fanatic who is mad about God, or the dictator who is mad about his own destructive omnipotence.

Denial and infantile sexual theories are normal and even desirable in children, for they are the breeding ground of infantile sexuality which persists in us, in the magma of our unconscious minds until the end of our days.

Gender theories

In adults, however, denial and childhood sexual theories can take a more pathological turn, culminating in forms of behaviour such as fetishism or delusional constructions.

What is "gender"? First of all, it is a word. A word that, alongside masculine/feminine, introduces a third gender into French, one that does not exist in our language: the neuter. *Ne-uter*, in Latin, means neither one nor the other. According to Judith Butler, this word means that the difference between the sexes is nothing more than a social norm imposed by the heterosexual hegemony, that it implies a relationship of domination, and that women are an invention of macho men. There is no longer anything biological or anatomical; no longer opposing sexes, but multiple genders. The proposal is to challenge and subvert theories of the anatomical difference between the sexes, including any binary concept. Hence Monique Wittig's dictum: "Lesbians are not women."

Social debates therefore focus on multiple gender differences, but not sexual differences. It may be said, then, that gender theories provide adults with a function that is identical to infantile sexual theories. But what is their fate when they go so far as to deny the anatomical difference between the sexes, and become part of a belief system, an ideology concerning identity itself? What traumatic force could have given rise to such a massive defence as that of the construction of "Queer theory" which considers that we have the right to proclaim ourselves to be men if we were born women, women if we were born men, and to say that we belong to either gender or are neither one nor the other.

The parents of a Swedish child, who refused to reveal his sex to him, declared: "We want Pop to grow up freely, and not in the mould of a specific gender." It is to be hoped that Pop will was able to experience the shock of the perception of the anatomical difference between the sexes, described by Freud as traumatic, and above all that he was able to construct his own infantile sexual theories. "Even if we see you naked," says a teacher, "we won't be able tell if you're male or female. Your inner sex doesn't necessarily correspond to your outer sex."

Some people do not fit into these gender theories. These are people born with an indeterminate sex, hermaphrodites or "transsexuals" who suffer from the painful conviction that they have suffered a biological error or sexual assignment. Since they do not depend on self-determination, they are people to be respected and approached with caution and sensitivity.

The social and political debates that inform these positions, which are particularly heated at the moment, tend to place them outside the intrapsychic conflict. These gender theories want to ignore what is essential in mental life: the fact that the sexual register is traumatic, that there is no desire or satisfaction without anxiety, that sexual drives are constant, excessive, impossible to satisfy fully, and that the ego must deploy all its defences to avoid being overwhelmed by them. Identificatory and fantasy-based movements and their unconscious aspects are ignored or denied.

A recent questionnaire given to 3rd Grade pupils, i.e. aged 14, was worded as follows

Sex: – Male – Female – Other.

Fortunately, the Ministry of Education was able to intervene and the term "Other" was removed.

A current phenomenon, both epidemic and ideological, concerns the demand for "sexual transition," that is a sex change, on the part of adolescents of both sexes. It is a matter of grave concern that doctors are using hormonal blockades or that surgeons are amputating sexual organs without any in-depth study of the underlying unconscious psychic terrain. The age of adolescence, a time of transition, is particularly a time of questioning about sexual identity and identifications. Responding to an experience of ill-being with an immediate and illusory solution that does not respect the time it takes for an adolescent to develop and grow physically and psychologically is an act fraught with serious consequences. Responding by concrete means, without considering the intrapsychic dimension, can have catastrophic consequences.[1]

Is it not the case that the demand for self-determination and the immediate response to it both reveal a fantasy of omnipotence? A form of triumph over the ordeal of the primal scene and the wound of Oedipal renunciation? A fantasy of self-procreation? Is this not a way of escaping the fatality of having only one sex, of experiencing a lack, of lacking the other sex? Of being dependent on sexuality? And sometimes of confusing identity with the choice of object, when in fact the affirmation of "transidentity" can simply lead to the discovery of an unacceptable homosexual tendency? The latest delusion, driven by computer technology, goes so far as to advocate "asexuality," a form of remote sexuality that avoids touching and therefore any contamination. "Yes, sex is dangerous, and desire is a fatally transmissible disease. The difference between the sexes is an incurable disease" (Schneider, 2007, p. 127).

This confirms the idea that what does violence to the ego, both individual and social, and to its narcissism, at any age, is the intrapsychic conflict of the difference between the sexes. For the ego has a narcissistic ideal of uniqueness, and this is threatened by difference, by otherness. Yet it is this conflict that contributes to the construction not only of psychosexuality, but of thought. Thought is to do with thinking about difference (Héritier, 1996).

Psychic bisexuality

Bisexuality, which is more narcissistic in essence, is situated on the side of primary or secondary identifications, while the elaboration of the difference between the sexes, which is more libidinal and object-related, is situated more on the side of erotic cathexes. Both concern the sexual identity of the subject and the choice of object.

Psychic bisexuality plays an essential organizing role in identifications, particularly in the crossed identifications of the Oedipal conflict.

However, fantasies of bisexuality, as well as acted-out bisexuality, can be a defence against working through the difference between the sexes, at the level of cathecting sexual otherness and genital sexual relations. Above all, it is a question of maintaining the possibility of being everything and having everything, an ideal that harks back to infantile omnipotence.

Nowadays, there is a tendency to exalt acted-out bisexuality, to the point of claiming that it represents progress in sexuality and that it is the future of humanity. Today's teenagers do not hesitate to ask questions such as: "Are you straight, gay or bisexual"? Personally, I think that this is still a form of repudiating or refusing to accept the feminine sphere.

Note

1 The "La petite sirène Observatoire" warns of the increase in consultations for gender dysphoria among children and adolescents. See Caroline Eliacheff and Céline Masson (2022).

References

André, J. (1995). *Aux origines féminines de la sexualité*. Paris: Presses Universitaires de France.
André, J. (2019). Sexualités, diversités. Internet site *Les enfants de la psychanalyse*, article dated 13 September.
Eliacheff, C., & Masson, C (2022). *La fabrique de l'enfant transgenre*. Paris: Les éditions de l'Observatoire.
Freud, S. (1912). On the universal tendency to debasement in the sphere of love (contributions to the psychology of love, II). *S.E.* 11. London: Hogarth, pp. 179–190.
Freud, S. (1915). Instincts and their vicissitudes. *S.E.* 14. London: Hogarth, pp. 117–140.
Freud, S. (1917). On transformations of instinct as exemplified in anal erotism. *S.E.* 17. London: Hogarth, pp. 127–133.
Freud, S. (1923). The infantile genital organization. *S.E.* 19. London: Hogarth, pp. 141–145.
Freud, S. (1933 [1932]). Femininity. In: *New Introductory Lectures on Psychoanalysis*. *S.E.* 22. London: Hogarth, pp. 112–132.
Guignard, F. (1997). Épitre à l'objet. Paris: Presses Universitaires de France.
Héritier, F. (1996). *Masculin/féminin, la pensée de la différence*. Paris: Odile Jacob.
Lacan, J. (1977/1963). *The Four Fundamental Concepts of Psychoanalysis*, trans. Alan Sheridan. London: Hogarth.
Schneider, M. (2007). *La confusion des sexes*. Paris: Flammarion.
Winnicott, D. (1971). The split off male and female elements to be found clinically in men and women. In: *Playing and Reality*. London: Tavistock, pp. 72–85.

Chapter 3

Preludes to the feminine sphere

How do girls become aware of the feminine sphere?

Was a child wanted? Did the parents want a girl? Recognition begins at the moment of birth. The child carries the projection of the parents' narcissism, which constitutes and nourishes its primary narcissism, the omnipotent narcissism of "His majesty the baby," and then its ego ideal.

Primary maternal impregnation

What is at play at the dawn of life is the antagonism and alternation between the mother's erotic and maternal cathexes.

Freud theorized that there is both an exemplary primary identification with the father of the child's prehistory and a primary identification that is indistinguishable from an initial cannibalistic oral cathexis. The aim, for the child, is to become completely at one with the mother, where "being" and "having" are indistinguishable. Freud expresses it thus: "I am the breast."

When this identification has been experienced with mutual happiness, in the sensual and narcissistic fusional honeymoon, it provides the fantasy of a lost paradise retrospectively. This, however, is on the condition that "defusion" has occurred owing to the progressive alternation of the mother's presence/absence, thereby permitting the hallucination of satisfaction and the onset of auto-erotic activities, the very first mental activities of the young infant.

A satisfactory primary identification is the cradle of the future maternal capacities of the little girl and later of the woman once she has become a mother, as well as those of the little boy and the future father. In this identification, where there is as yet no differentiation, the archaic fantasies of being eaten up, of being engulfed again in the maternal womb, a prelude to the inescapable defusion, can be processed by the child if the mother is able to "contain" (in Bion's sense) all these movements. Children's stories provide a precious means of helping the child to process these first fantasies, through the figures of the wolf, the ogre and the ogress.

If this mode of primary identification has not taken place, if the paternal function is inoperative, if the mother has not been able to cathect her child or if she has over-cathected him or her to complete herself narcissistically,

DOI: 10.4324/9781003471042-3

leaving them no space of lack to hallucinate, the child cannot differentiate the parental images or elaborate their primal fantasies of the primal scene and castration. They remain attached to a figure of "combined parents," to use Melanie Klein's expression. The child may construct a threatening and dangerous world with these same fantasies, which are then psychotic anxieties and constitute attempts at self-healing through visual representation. They cannot easily be elaborated through stories or games.

This zone of the ego, a zone of disquieting strangeness, which lies within each of us, is always open. It has a potential for regressive attraction that can always be reactivated in the event of conflicts of identification or drive-related conflicts. In certain moments of analytic treatment, this zone can generate fantasies of fusional narcissistic omnipotence, and its deadly reverse side: anxieties about psychic death, monstrous figures of combined parents, pregenital incest and annihilating re-engulfment in the maternal body.

Moreover, if this primary identification was unsatisfactory or incomplete, it will be perpetuated by the compulsion to repeat in a never-ending quest for a fusional relationship, or in a repetition of the identical.

The constitution of the primeval fantasy of the primal scene is a pivotal moment in extricating the subject from the relationship to this *imago* of the archaic mother. It is the crucible of all the alternating identifications of the Oedipal organization, and of the erotic cathexes questioning the enigma of the difference between the sexes.

The mother, the first seductress

Freud (1933) refers to the awakening of the erogenous zones by maternal care, which "touches the ground of reality" (p. 120).

The first extraction of the sexual drives based on, and in opposition to, the supporting system of self-preservative needs, can be inferred from this. The nurturing breast gives way to an erotic breast, providing itself and the infant with a satisfaction that, according to Freud, is the prototype of the satisfaction of orgasm in love.

The primary bond with the mother, the care-giving mother and the seductive mother, enables the infant to have two fundamental experiences: enjoyment in passivity and dependence on the other in the search for and discovery of pleasure. Through her gaze, voice, gestures and words, a mother awakens the erotization of the child's body, awakens its erogenous zones, and lets herself be seduced by the infant with whom she has pleasure.

In his theory of "generalized primal seduction," Jean Laplanche (1989/1987) takes into account the mother's unconscious, in the sense that she offers the infant enigmatic verbal and non-verbal signifiers imbued with unconscious sexual meanings. The enigma for the infant, according to him, could be formulated as follows: "What does this breast that excites itself by suckling me want from me?" But the infant at the breast also seduces the mother, and the enigmatic message (according to Laurence Kahn) could be formulated as follows: "What does this shameless, cannibalistic, homosexual, incestuous child want from me?" This is a fitting reversal of what was originally an emergence of the mother's own unconscious activity with the child, even though she was unaware of it. It has even been described as a situation of "primordial incest" (Cabrol, 2011).

But it is important that the exciting mother is able to provide the child with anti-cathexes to her excess of excitation by also acting as a stimulus barrier. For the baby girl, the outline of the feminine sphere is formed when the mother returns to her sexual night. When she rediscovers her erotic life as a woman, by inciting her baby to sleep, she is no longer a mother and exercises a censorship, known as the "censorship of the woman-as-lover (*censure de l'amante*)" (Braunschweig & Fain, 1975).

This consists in transmitting to her child, through her own body, a mediated message designating an "other" of her desire, enabling the child to organize his or her excitation towards an "other," as a prelude to the construction of an object and to subsequent triangulation

It is by virtue of this censorship governing the sleep/dream system and this alternation that the mother can protect her baby from all forms of erotic desire: her desire for her infant, the father/lover's desire for her, and her desire for the father's penis. There is an alternation between the post-Oedipal baby of daytime reality and the hallucinatory, pregenital or Oedipal baby of the night.

The aim of this censorship is also to protect her baby from confusion at the level of its erotic impulses and to shelter it from its own sexual ecstasy. It is therefore desexualizing for her baby and resexualizing for her lover. This alternation, both physical and mental, of the mother's absence, also enables the infant to create its first mental proto-organizations, those of autoeroticism and the hallucination of satisfaction. It thus facilitates the libidinal development and efflorescence not only of the infant, but also of the mother, who can alternate sexual relations and maternal care, reviving fully her infantile sexuality, without the burden of guilt for betraying and abandoning the child, and without blurring erotic sensations.

By remaining silent about the erogeneity of the little girl's genitals, the mother establishes a "primary repression of the vagina." This allows a girl's entire body to develop diffuse erotic capacities, in anticipation of her awakening to the revelation of her own genitals by the lover of ecstatic pleasure. The tale of "Sleeping Beauty," whose sexual organs are dormant, offers an age-old illustration of this.

The manner in which the infant experiences this seduction by the mother, and infant's release from it, with the support of the father figure, will determine the future of their erotic life.

Maternal seduction does not only excite the erotogenic zones; it also stimulates the infant's ability to react to effects of surprise. For example, by playing "peek-a-boo" games. If the mother reassures the infant by holding it close to her and laughing, it can then laugh with her. This seduction helps the infant to get used to the sudden irruption of what is new, foreign, unexpected and destabilizing, where the possibility of trauma lies. It contains the increased excitation in a space of play, which will enable the infant to make the journey of transforming excitation into drive activity, until it can create its own game, the wooden reel game. The mother is both exciting and acts as a stimulus barrier.

Early maternal seduction is therefore an apprenticeship in the drive and the object. It is an initiatory experience. The father's seduction, opening up a breach, will be its deferred effect. Early seduction is part of an organizing movement of the psyche and of infantile sexuality, while the subsequent seduction reveals the success or failure of this organization.

In the mutual seduction between the infant and its mother, there is an exchange of looks in which the promise to be what satisfies the desire of the other can be read. The impossibility of this wish means that the promise inherent in any form of seduction cannot be kept. It leads fatally to disappointment and disillusionment. If the emergence of sexuality inflicts a narcissistic wound on every human being, the infinite hope of reparation raised by seduction is doomed to inevitable disappointment. The father's penetrating seduction is structuring subsequently, in the sense that it allows for the disillusionment of omnipotence and the advent of castration anxiety, which organizes the Oedipus complex.

Derived from Freud's work with hysterics, the concept of seduction is fundamentally linked to that of trauma, but once Freud had abandoned his *neurotica*, the actual scene of traumatic seduction, the effect of seduction became generalizable to any increase in excitation, whether linked to a fantasy, producing internal excitation, or provoked by external excitation reactivating the unconscious scenario.

What can a mother pass on to her daughter?

A mother can pass on femininity. Femininity is the body, appearance, lure, masquerade, the charming accessories of seduction – dresses, heels, jewellery – that go hand in with the phallic dimension.

In a relationship of love, tenderness and complicity, a mother can pass on to her daughter all the trappings of femininity. If she lends herself to it and accepts the identification, she can pass on the charm of seduction towards men, and even the desire for a loving relationship, provided that the parental couple shows signs of it. This femininity can be passed on from mother to daughter and also from daughter to mother! Provided that is, that a generational difference is respected through identification, and not mimicry, a mirror relationship or sisterhood as is the case with mothers who act like little girls or little girls who act like young women!

A little girl who puts her little feet into her mother's high-heeled shoes knows that it's a game, and quickly goes back to playing in her trainers. An adolescent girl, depending on the nature of her Oedipal rivalry, may adopt a provocative exhibitionist attitude, or shun femininity and dress like a sack of potatoes. But if the mother is envious, she may wear the same miniskirts and jewellery as her daughter, or even seduce her friends. She can also do everything she can to make her daughter unalluring: "Mirror, my beautiful mirror"! We know the answer.

The feminine sphere, however, cannot be passed on from mother to daughter. If femininity is the body, the feminine sphere is the flesh, and it is the erotic dimension of the flesh. It is interior, invisible and disquieting, bearing "anxieties related to the feminine sphere" (Schaeffer, 1997) in both sexes.

If the mother has not given her daughter a penis, which, according to Freud, turns her into an object of hatred, she does not give her a vagina either. Nor can she pass on to her the feminine sphere.

A daughter can only become a woman if she can *resist* her mother's maternal feminine sphere. A certain degree of antagonism seems necessary for elaborating certain phases in the development of the little girl's libido, in conformity with her mother's maternal and erotic feminine dimension. This is the fantasy of the mother and the whore. A little girl may one day violently reject her mother's affectionate caresses, thereby manifesting the deferred effect of maternal seduction and the incestuous nature of pregenital relationships. Separating from the mother, losing her, implies thinking of her as a woman and entering into the Oedipal situation. The daughter now turns towards her father. Hand-play with her mother has now become "naughty" play (Schaeffer, 2002).

Too much of the maternal dimension, aimed at excluding the paternal figure and using the daughter as a narcissistic complement, may lead to very serious disturbances in the daughter's sense of identity and future sexuality as a woman. But too much of the lover in the mother could give rise in the daughter to a hatred of the woman-as-lover, of the primal scene and sexuality, leading potentially to severe hysteria, frigidity and frequent somatic decompensations.

Some mothers can also pass on to their daughters their hatred of men, their devaluation, terror and horror of the penis, and their distaste for the sexual act and penetration, which may turn a girl towards various forms of homosexuality.

The messenger of expectant waiting

What a mother can pass on to her daughter is above all a capacity for expectant waiting. This capacity is nourished by receptiveness towards the surge of the drives, the "choreography of the encounter," maternal seduction, and the "primary mirror" function. In other words, everything that the mother's face can mirror and duplicate to the little girl concerning her quest for an image of herself, her sensations, affects and drive processes (Roussillon, 2011). It is nourished by transmission through speech, tender words, the words of childhood that the mother discovers again, to which the little girl responds by babbling, words that will forever infuse its vocal style during loving relationships, its first childhood loves, but also those of adolescence or even adulthood.

The good enough mother knows how to rhythm her absences and returns so that the period of waiting is neither too short nor too long for the infant. She allows the infant to organize itself mentally, through the hallucination of satisfaction and autoeroticism, until it is able to create an internal object that binds the anxiety of separation. She is thus a messenger of expectant waiting.

From the very beginning, the way a mother cathects a boy or a girl narcissistically or erotically is not the same. The boy can satisfy his so-called phallic narcissism more easily, whereas the girl – of the same sex as her and the same sex as her own mother – can arouse in her either feelings of rivalry or anxieties to do with the fantasy of female "castration," as well as other more archaic anxieties, those of feminine sexual ecstasy and incest (Schaeffer, 2006). True incest always involves the mother, and is linked to returning to the mother's womb. Incest between mother and daughter has been seen as the fundamental homosexual fantasy.

It is the mother who sexualizes waiting by means of the censorship of the lover, and who makes the child suffer the discontinuous pain of maternal decathexis, when the lover is no longer a mother. It is the connection between erotic excitation and the pain of this discontinuous loss of the primary maternal object that definitively includes sexual desire in this cathexis of the relationship between sexual ecstasy and pain. All this comes under the seal of primary masochism. It is therefore the mother who determines the quality of the fusion of the drives.

If the Beauty is to fall asleep peacefully, protected by the primary repression of her vagina, she must be able to cathect expectant waiting. If the mother, the messenger of castration according to Freud, says to the little boy who rushes forward with his penis at the ready: "Be careful, or you'll get into trouble," she says to her daughter: "Wait and see, one day your Prince Charming will come!" She is thus the messenger of expectant waiting. In most cases, then, she subjects the girl to phallic, symbolic logic, to the law of the father.

Boys are destined in principle for a sexuality of conquest, of penetration. Grounded in their anality and castration anxiety, they usually organize themselves in terms of activity and the control of waiting. Whereas girls, women, are destined to wait: first they wait for a penis, then breasts and "periods," the first time, and then every month thereafter; they wait for penetration, pregnancy, childbirth, weaning and so on. They are always waiting… For the most part, these times of waiting are linked to uncontrollable experiences of real losses of parts of themselves or their objects. Since girls, unlike boys, are unable to symbolize them as anxiety related to losing an organ – which is rarely lost in reality – and are subject to upheavals in their narcissistic economy, they need to be firmly anchored to primary masochism (Rosenberg, 1991). This makes it possible to cathect painful tension erotically, to tolerate the frustration caused by the non-satisfaction of the drives which, by nature, are impossible to satisfy, as well as the discrepancy between hallucinatory wish-fulfilment and the expectation of real satisfaction, and subsequently to experience the pleasure/pain of sexual ecstasy.

This does not prevent little girls from developing all sorts of infantile sexual theories, and fantasizing that everything would be better if they had a penis. In fact, this penis is above all a phallus, in other words the narcissistic over-valuing that is accorded to it. The fantasy that what they lack will "grow" later sets them on the path of waiting for the person who will replace their missing penis with a baby. For Freud, the desire for a child precedes erotic desire.

This, Freud says, is how the change of object begins, and how the girl, disappointed by her mother, turns to the father.

Freeing oneself from the mother

What is deeply terrifying, for both sexes, is the proximity of the mother's sexual organ from which they came. This greed of the drive pressure, always unsatisfied, is terrifying if it harks back to fears of being eaten up, engulfed in the mother's body, the object of terror and the lost paradise of fusion/confusion.

An *imago* is an internalized figure, often tyrannical in its demands. Freeing itself from the mother's ascendancy is what the child tried to do during the phallic phase. This phase, in which the penis is hypercathected narcissistically, is an obligatory passage for both girls and boys, because it is one of the means of freeing themselves from the pregenital *imago* and maternal influence.

Etymologically speaking: sex (from the Latin *sectus*) is what splits, cuts, separates. The fact that little boys have a visible penis enables them to separate and differentiate themselves from their mother. It signifies a limit, a difference, leading to the representation of the sexual organs and the difference between the sexes, and thus serves as a support of symbolization. Boys, in principle, have the means to free themselves from the mother because they have a penis that the mother does not have; and also because, thanks to their paternal identification, they can negotiate, via castration anxiety, the symbolization of the part for the whole. In principle, boys are prepared for a sexuality of conquest, that is, of penetration.

But what about an erotic feminine dimension? The negotiation of the part for the whole seems problematic. This is why anal representations of what comes out, of what can be lost but also renewed, like faeces, caught in the chain of transpositions, as well as phallic representations of castration and penis envy, can represent good symbolic defences for girls and women against their anxiety related to the feminine sphere, or concerning things that get inside and are invasive. The change of object to a father who has a penis and who can separate her from the pregenital mother enables the daughter to cathect the father's penis and the fantasy of the child he is expected to give her, etc. But a child from the father remains in the phallic-anal line of descent as a gift, a substitute object, and it is therefore still only a question of what I shall call a "work of femininity."

The fact remains that the interior and everything that gets inside it must also be symbolized. This is the "work of the feminine sphere" that has to be accomplished throughout a woman's life, in parallel with the symbolic working-through of losses of part-objects, carried out, as for men, on what is visible and on the body of the other.

The destiny of the girl's attachment to her mother

The girl's dependence on the archaic pre-Oedipal mother, the so-called Mino-Mycenaean period, lasts for a period that Freud admits he had underestimated for a long time: "A number of women remain arrested in their original attachment to their mother and never achieve a true change-over towards men" (Freud, 1931, p. 226).

The paradox of the feminine destiny lies in the difficulty of freeing oneself from a primary maternal object, due to a necessary identification and an equally necessary disidentification. Separation brings with it the risk of losing a part of oneself, and thus the onset of depressive feelings.

This is why a daughter's attachment to her mother is often one of love and hate. Lacan calls it a "ravage." But hatred allows for separation. The quality of the attachment lies in the predominance of one colour over the other, between red and black. But the attachment is indestructible, and manifests itself in all the registers of fidelity, for or against.

References

Braunschweig, D., & Fain, M. (1975). *La nuit, le jour. Essai psychanalytique sur le fonctionnement mental.* Paris: Presses Universitaires de France.

Cabrol, G. (2011). Le refoulement de l'inceste primordial. *Bulletin de la Société Psychanalytique de Paris*, 99: 99–103

Freud, S. (1931). Female sexuality. *S.E.* 21. London: Hogarth, pp. 225–243.

Freud, S. (1933). New Introductory Lectures to Psychoanalysis. *S.E.* 22. London: Hogarth, pp. 1–182.

Laplanche, J. (1989/1987). *New Foundations in Psychoanalysis,* trans. D. Mâcey. Oxford: Blackwell.

Rosenberg, B. (1991). Masochisme mortifère et masochisme gardien de vie. In: *Monographies de la Revue française de Psychanalyse*. Paris: Presses Universitaires de France, pp. 17–160.

Roussillon, R. (2011). Le concept du maternel primaire. *Le maternel, Revue française de psychanalyse*, 75(5): 1497–1504.

Schaeffer, J. (1997). Mal-être dans la sexualité. In: *Débats de psychanalyse, Le Mal-être (angoisse et violence)*. Paris: Presses Universitaires de France, pp. 89–100.

Schaeffer, J. (2002). Le parcours des antagonismes entre féminin et maternel. In: *La parentalité. Défi pour le troisième millénaire*. Paris: Presses Universitaires de France, pp. 139–155.

Schaeffer, J. (2006). Le tabou du féminin. In: *Monographies et Débats de Psychanalyse, Interdit et Tabou.* Paris: Presses Universitaires de France, pp. 171–191.

Chapter 4

Feminine sexuality

An endless story

> "The little girl is a little man."
>
> Freud (1933, p. 118)

Puberty. The emergence of the vagina

In adolescence, at puberty, both girls and boys are suddenly made aware of the emergence of the female sexual organ. Puberty generates an excessive influx of libidinal pressure. The identity-based ego and the defensive ego are in difficulty, and sometimes in danger. Internal excitation is constant. The irruption of the body into psychosexuality during puberty manifests itself both as a psychical breach and as a deferred process.

The great discovery of puberty, for both sexes, is that of the vagina. It is no longer the perception of the difference between the sexes and the enigma of the relationship between the parents that breaks through into consciousness, but the emergence of the feminine sphere, which can no longer be denied. Girls are no longer determined by a lack, but by the appearance of something more: they find that their breasts – rather than a penis – are growing, and their vagina appears. It is then the feminine component that appears as the extraneous element that causes a breach in the mind with the result that "Throne and Altar are in danger," as Freud puts it.

According to Freud, the vagina is still undiscovered during childhood by both sexes due to the intense narcissistic phallic cathexis of the penis, the only sexual organ of childhood. There is in fact no infantile organ. Little girls, of course, are perfectly aware that they have a hollowed-out area in their body. They feel internal sensations aroused by Oedipal impulses just as much as by the archaic traces of the body-to-body relationship with the primitive mother, the first seductress, according to Freud. However, the true revelation of the erotic vagina, the profound erogeneity of this female organ, can only be accomplished within sexual relations of ecstatic pleasure.

The awakening of puberty occurs long before the capacity for a sexual relationship is developed. As Winnicott suggests, sexual activity comes into

DOI: 10.4324/9781003471042-4

play more as a way of getting rid of sexuality than as an attempt to experience it. Castration anxiety linked to bodily transformations, the emergence of genitality, the sense of narcissistic incompleteness, and the confusion of *imagos* all reactivate anxieties to do with confusion with the maternal body, and the sexual relationship that has now become possible reawakens the fantasized danger of incest.

The fantasy of seduction can take on a persecutory character. The Oedipal conflict flares up again, and "anxieties related to the feminine sphere" must strive free themselves from pregenital anxieties. All these anxieties call for a differentiated readjustment of the *imagos* and require a new change of object. Adolescents must distance themselves from their parents, can no longer stand the cuddles and caresses they used to love, and the outside world makes them feel anxious. This can lead to defiant, contraphobic or withdrawn forms of behaviour, not to mention all the addictive and psychopathic behaviours, among others.

The emergence of the feminine sphere at puberty changes the nature of the castration complex. Castration anxiety is compounded by penetration anxiety, in both sexes, well beyond the anxiety about losing the penis, or about not having one.

This is the big question of adolescence: how can the fantasies generated by the discovery of this new organ, the vagina, be processed? How do boys use their penis for sexual fulfilment? How do they encounter the feminine component, which is no longer the absence of a penis, but another sexual organ? How do they deal with this anxiety! How do girls go through these bodily transformations that no longer refer to a lack, but to an expansion? And how can a girl tear herself away from the maternal imago, when her body begins to resemble her mother's body, sometimes even merging with it in fantasy? These transformations bring her dangerously close to the primal scene and incestuous enactment.

In girls, drive activity remains very close to the body, to the source. It is the womb, the inside of the body, which can be the object of anxiety, or threatened with destruction in fantasy, as Melanie Klein suggested. It is threatened more by invasion and intrusion than by what can be torn off or cut. A girl's pregenital intrusion anxieties will have to be transformed into penetration anxiety. The transition from pregenital intrusion anxieties to genital penetration anxieties is often marked by fantasies of rape.

The adolescent girl's sexual body may be experienced as an enemy, strange and abnormal. Conflicts of identification are involved. The gaze of others is sought as a vehicle for the quest for identity, and the reflection of the self-image is both intensely expected and violently rejected by the adolescent, who is both seeking recognition and identification and demanding de-identification.

Those girls who have been the most cuddly and affectionate may feel disgust for their mother's body and reject any form of bodily contact and seduction. Freud's (1919) analysis of the fantasy "A child is being beaten" revealed that the deeply repressed feminine Oedipal desire for the father could only be satisfied through masochism. How can a girl approach the real father other than by letting herself be mistreated by him and by provoking him? How can she fail to flee from him?

It is during adolescence, when sexual penetration and the erotic vagina are cathected, that deficiencies of internalization and dangers of narcissistic intrusion may reappear. Puberty then has a traumatic effect. For girls, it reactivates fears of intrusion and confusion with the maternal body, which can lead to eating disorders.

This reawakening during the second stage of the biphasism of human psychosexuality reactivates the Oedipal conflict and fears of incestuous relationships, and also causes narcissistic and identity-related disturbances. But this second stage may also allow for the retroactive reorganization of everything that could not be adequately processed during the Oedipal situation. Moreover, beyond the inevitable disturbances, the crisis may have a positive effect in bringing about a readjustment of cathexes and identifications.

The Oedipal organization in girls

The main organizer of the mind is the Oedipal conflict. Its orchestra director is castration anxiety, its inescapable prerequisite the phallic organization, and its culmination the elaboration of two differences: that of the sexes and that of the generations.

Castration anxiety, the central operator of the Oedipal conflict, presides over the phallic organization, which stems from an infantile sexual theory, that of the narcissistic over-valuation of a single sexual organ, the penis, erected as a phallus, glorified and even deified in certain civilizations. It is an all-or-nothing mode of defence that consists in denying the difference between the sexes, and therefore the feminine sphere, equated with "castration." The feminine sphere is what is problematic for the difference between the sexes.

This organization, however, is a necessary stage for both sexes, because it allows them to free themselves from the pregenital *imago* of the omnipotent mother and maternal influence. The father's symbolic phallic function establishes the law, which enables the father to separate the child from the mother and bring the child into the social world. We know just how far this function is essential and endangered today.

The outcome of the Oedipus complex differs depending on one's sex. In principle, a boy is favoured by the fact that he has a penis that his mother does not have. Thanks to his castration anxiety, he can symbolize the part for the whole, supported by his paternal identification. In principle, he renounces his incestuous wishes violently: he enters the phallic phase and renounces the whole in order to save the part, to save his penis, under the threat of castration anxiety.

But what about an erotic feminine sphere? Since it is difficult to negotiate the part for the whole, how can a girl be recognized as a sexual being in the absence of the penis she perceives as the bearer of all narcissistic value? How can she symbolize an inside that is a whole, and how can she separate her own inside from her mother's? Can the female sexual organs be symbolized and rendered psychically operative?

Her unconscious ploy will be to erase this problematic difference and adopt the phallic logic. Penis envy is narcissistic, not erotic, because the girl may well feel that this lack does not prevent her from having access to all sorts of voluptuous sensations. And she is well aware, unconsciously, that autoeroticism is the object of a conflict, which is linked to the parental objects.

Freud claims that girls do not experience castration anxiety because this is already accomplished. This is obviously nothing more than a fantasy (but it does raise questions about the existence of Freud's theory of infantile sexuality). Freud speaks of a castration complex in girls, and therefore of a structural operator, the Oedipus complex, which organizes the difference between the sexes and the generations of both sexes. Ideally, according to Freud, both sexes will only free themselves from the phallic/castrated pairing at puberty, before coming to terms with the masculine/feminine pairing, that of the difference between the sexes.

In *Inhibitions,* Symptoms and Anxiety, Freud (1926) describes the process of integrating anxieties to do with loss in terms of situations of danger. This process goes from anxieties about losing everything to anxieties about partial losses. The castration complex reorganizes after the event all the earlier archaic anxieties to do with loss, which have already been subject to a defensive organization based on the active/passive pairing. Freud (1917) had already set out this anal logic of organ equivalences and partial losses in an article. The castration anxiety of the phallic phase can only be reassured by the equivalence of the loss of the penis and the loss of excrement, since this is an operation that can be controlled by the anal sphincter, and of a part-object whose return is guaranteed, periodically. Unless, that is, a child is psychotic.

Freud contrasts castration anxiety in men with separation anxiety, loss of object and loss of love in women. A girl's anxiety is therefore not about castration, but about the loss of love. Rather than the loss of a part, underpinning the capacity for symbolization, it is the loss of the whole that she is threatened with, the whole of the cathexis of her body, and the whole of her object, the whole of being more than the whole of having (Schaeffer, 2013). Hence women's propensity for depression. This is why anal representations of what comes out, of what can be lost, but also renewed, caught in the chain of transpositions of the drives (Freud, 1917), phallic representations of castration and penis envy, can represent good symbolic defences for girls and women against their anxieties related to the feminine sphere, against anxiety about what is lost, but also of what gets inside and is invasive.

Castration anxiety is coupled with penetration anxiety, in both sexes, but asymmetrically, signifying difference. The phallic/castrated pairing must evolve towards the construction of a masculine/feminine pairing.

The change of object

Freud's theory that the little girl is a "little man" until puberty has been a source of discussion and controversy, and the question has still not been resolved. Freud speaks of the need for a change of object so that the little girl can develop from being a "little man" into a woman.

Since the mother has not given her daughter a penis, which, according to Freud, earns her the most hateful reproaches, the daughter will turn towards her father for recognition. This is what leads her into the Oedipal conflict. She enters it, according to Freud, to acquire a penis, thanks to her father, who will later give her a child as a substitute for the penis, and she leaves it with difficulty, sometimes never, because of her mother. I am exaggerating, of course.

While the castration complex can have a structuring and symbolizing value, it is only insofar as it allows access to the recognition of the paternal penis as a separator from the pregenital attachment to the mother.

The father's recognition of his daughter's femininity is essential. It is this recognition that establishes a difference with the mother's "mirror" gaze, according to Winnicott (1971), directing the daughter towards another gaze, one that will leave its mark on the destiny of the woman's femininity in the sense of wanting to be looked at and desired by a man. I mean the father's gaze which intimates "You're a pretty little girl," but also, in an Oedipal anti-incestuous register, "One day your prince will come along." This paternal cathexis is what can prevent the depressive risk entailed by the sense of lacking a sexual organ, or of having a castrated organ.

But is it simply a matter of expecting a baby from the father in fantasy, as reparation for the slight of not having received a penis from the mother, in order to fulfil herself narcissistically? Or is it more a question of waiting to be recognized and loved erotically? Female erotic desires for the father are not mentioned by Freud, for whom the desire for a child precedes erotic desire.

What characterizes the feminine Oedipus is a movement of reversal from activity to active passivity characterized by the feminine masochistic movement (Parat, 1995a). In other words, a shift, towards the father, of a masochistic movement addressed to the mother, so that everything that happens to the girl's sexual body can be expected and attributed to the man's penis. This change of object of the cathexis of waiting and masochism is what will facilitate an evolution towards the male/female pairing of the erotic encounter.

The feminine sphere and femininity in both sexes

Femininity is to do with the body. The feminine is to do with the flesh. It is the interior, what is invisible and disturbing, generating anxiety in both sexes.

Femininity in a woman is appearance, masquerade, the charming accessories of seduction – dresses, high heels, jewellery, make-up – which matches well with the phallic organization.

It is with regard to her anxiety about an internal female sex organ that is invisible and unrepresentable that a girl, a woman, has recourse to cathecting femininity. If a man narcissistically overvalues his penis, a woman cathects her entire body, but it remains tied to the reassurance of the other's gaze.

This visible femininity goes hand-in-hand with phallic logic. It consists in valuing, according to the same model, what is seen, what is shown and exhibited, and what externalizes itself, and has the aim of reassuring castration anxiety in both men and women.

These visible aspects of femininity are in fact a veil concealing the unformed, elusive, unrepresentable hollow of the female sex, its disturbing openness, its overflowing fluids, the blood that escapes from it. The exaltation of feminine curves, of the exquisite shape of the breast, counter-cathects this anxiety aroused by formlessness. Phallic claims, in both men and women, are a defence against castration anxiety.

Femininity in a man manifests itself through the seduction of the body and its envelopes, whether they are sartorial or artistic. Men's homosexuality is the most obvious example of this. Fashion artists know how to shape the image that will be the object of a man's desire.

The feminine sphere, in a woman, on the sexual level, is what allows the recognition of the female sexual organ, when it is revealed through its access to ecstatic sexual pleasure.

From a metapsychological point of view, it is the capacity of a woman's ego to allow itself to be penetrated by large quantities of unbound excitation, without suffering a traumatic breach, and to be nourished and amplified by them.

This capacity of the feminine sphere sustains sexual ecstatic pleasure, but also the highly energetic bodily experiences of the maternal dimension in women, such as pregnancy, childbirth, as well as their psychic experiences.

The feminine sphere in a man, his "work on his feminine sphere," consists in allowing himself to be dominated by the constant libidinal pressure. It is the ability to relinquish, for a while, the control of his ego, to abandon his anal and phallic defences, to overcome the fantasies of a penis that tends above all to verify its solidity in the sexual relationship, and not to be terrorized by fantasies linked to the danger of the body of the woman/mother.

It is to enter into resonance with a woman's feminine sphere. Acknowledging this dimension of the feminine sphere in himself would provoke his drives to conquer those of a woman, sometimes even to lead her to discover them, reducing the split between affectionate and sensual currents, between mother and whore. It would also mean being able to maintain his desire for a single woman. As Michelet wrote in his *Journal,* "The sea and my wife's cunt are my two infinities!"

With another man, the feminine sphere, in identification with a woman, would consist in experiencing vast quantities of unbound excitation in a homosexual relationship.

The phallic function in both sexes

Many women have recently spoken out, and rightly so, when they have been the objects of sexual predators, humiliated, devalued and forced into submission.

From a psychoanalytical point of view, the domination of men, which is undeniable in the organization of all societies, refers to the necessary symbolic and phallic function of the father, which establishes the law and enables the father to separate the child from its mother and to facilitate its access to the social world.

It is disturbing to note the extent to which this "refusal of the feminine sphere" constitutes a general law of human behaviour and plays a part in the elaboration of their psychic genesis, to the point that Freud developed a phallocentric theory of psycho-sexual development, and Lacan made the phallus the central signifier of sexuation, desire and ecstatic pleasure. This observation helps us to understand the extent to which this infantile sexual theory – that there is only one sex organ, the phallic penis – may have constituted an energetic defensive tactic to defend against the traumatic upheaval caused by the discovery of the difference between the sexes, inaugurating the Oedipal organization. As can be seen in the social domain, it insists on maintaining it.

While it is undeniable that this domination is exercised predominantly by men, and that it rightly serves to stigmatize a certain form of patriarchy, it is important not to equate the masculine with the phallic, without giving the slightest consideration to the fact that it might be its antagonist! The phallic costume suits both genders equally well. However, the masculine/feminine pairing is a co-creation, which is contradiction with that of the phallic/castrated hierarchical order.

What really attacks the feminine sphere is not the masculine sphere, but the "phallic" sphere. In other words, the narcissistic, rather than erotic, hypercathexis of the male sexual organs, and the need to prove one's virility.

The masculine sphere refers to the feminine sphere, the phallic sphere forms a pair with what is "castrated," i.e. with sexual organs that are denied, belittled and despised: the female sexual organs. Harassing sexual predators, using power and violence, are not worthy of wearing the insignia of the "masculine" sphere.

The sexual drive is impetuous and wild. It is to be hoped that women will not deprive themselves of the gaze of men's desire, provided that they acknowledge their femininity and continue to hope to fulfil their feminine component. In respect of otherness, the most magnificent gift is that of ecstatic sexual pleasure.

Far from abolishing the mystery of the difference between the sexes, it merely exalts it. This is because it is based on the deepest level of human beings, namely, the survival of infantile sexuality, which leads to tireless curiosity about the nature of the most enigmatic sex of all: the female sex.

The phallic dimension is not the exclusive preserve of men; it manifests itself just as much in women. It drives the thirst for power, control and domination. It is the antagonist of power, in both men and women. The phallic affirmation, in both sexes, is a defence against castration anxiety. When this phallic affirmation is exacerbated, it can lead to a hypertrophy of the ego which becomes pathologized in the direction of paranoia. In some women, phallic affirmation can take over their femininity, at the expense of their feminine component and of their acknowledgement of the masculine component in men. It can also take the form of female hysteria.

A woman's feminine power is her desire to be desired. When she is not desired, or is no longer desired, she may feel deprived of her sexual organs. This may give rise to female castration anxiety, which concerns a woman's body and its capacity to attract, unlike male castration anxiety, which is anchored in a man's penis and its performance.

Penis envy and phallic affirmation

It is important to distinguish between penis envy and phallic affirmation. Phallic affirmation is narcissistic, and is defined as the narcissistic over-valuation of the penis.

Phallic affirmation initially concerns an omnipotent anal phallic mother, constituted as an *imago*, and can represent an almost insurmountable bedrock because the object of envy is an uncastratable anal phallus/penis that will be projected onto any person endowed with phallic power.

Penis envy, however, is directed at a genital mother who did not give her daughter a penis, and who is subsequently blamed for all the grievances possible. This envy conceals the desire for the object of the mother's desire: that is, the penis-bearing father.

This transition from the phallus to the penis, if I may say so, can take place in an atmosphere of intense guilt. One of my patients, after six years of analysis, following a dream in which she gave birth to a male child, talked to me about a capital offence, about high treason; she had the feeling that she was caught up in two contradictory movements and wanted to have it both ways. Another patient, who was unable to make this transition, felt trapped in a relationship between daughter and mother, and between mother and daughter with her child. She said: "It's like Russian dolls, we're all interlocked and can't get out; men at least have the certainty of being separated from their mother because they're not made like her."

Lacan claimed, apparently, that three categories of people were unanalysable, because of their overly direct or unsymbolizable relationship to the body, jouissance and death: women, priests and the Japanese (he'd seen the 1976 film, *Empire of the Senses*).

In the *Encyclopedia Universalis*, in the article "Féminité," M.M. (Michèle Montrelay, 1977) writes:

> A woman's speech can only be understood as an extension of her body; nothing is latent, everything is manifest. Femininity defeats analysis insofar as it overlooks repression and threatens representation. The continent is dark because it is out of the loop, foreclosed from the symbolic economy. A woman enjoys her body as she would the body of another person, her mother in particular. Women's archaic sexuality blocks symbolic castration.

Elsewhere, she writes: "The only salvation for women is through sublimation: women must revel in metaphor and jouissance must become writing."

Catherine Parat (1995b), moreover, uses the term "feminine phallic sphere" to refer to the domain of the different sublimations achieved thanks to the various feminine and virile identifications, and to the use of psychic bisexuality.

References

Freud, S. (1917). On transformations of instinct as exemplified in anal erotism. *S.E.* 17. London: Hogarth, pp. 127–133.

Freud, S. (1919). New Introductory Lectures to Psychoanalysis. *S.E.* 17. London: Hogarth, pp. 179–204.

Freud, S. (1926). Inhibitions, symptoms and anxiety. *S.E.* 20. London: Hogarth, pp. 75–175.

Freud, S. (1933 [1932]). Femininity. *S.E.* 22. London: Hogarth, pp. 112–135.

Montrelay, M. (1977). *L'ombre et le nom, Sur la féminité*. Paris: Éditions de Minuit.

Parat, C. (1995a). *L'affect partagé, Le fait psychanalytique*. Paris: Presses Universitaires de France.

Parat, C. (1995b). Le phallique féminin. *Revue française de psychanalyse,* 59(4): 1239–1257.

Schaeffer, J. (2013). Le risque de la perte. Angoisses et dépression au féminin. In: *Monographies et Débats de Psychanalyse, La sexualité féminine*. Paris: Presses Universitaires de France, pp. 110–128.

Winnicott, D.W. (1971). Mirror-role of mother and family in child development. In: *Playing and Reality*. London: Tavistock, pp. 111–118.

Chapter 5

Sexual and loving relationships

The encounter

> "I have been busy recently with a study of the sexual act, in the course of which I have discovered the pleasure pump ... as well as other *curiosa*, but for the time being I shall not talk about them."
>
> (Freud, Letter to Fliess dated 31 October 1895, in Masson, 1985, p. 148)

What about the question of the difference between the sexes in a relationship between a couple? I would say that it is not self-evident, and further that the feminine component, like the masculine component, at the genital level, is not something acquired at puberty, as Freud asserts, with the onset of the first sexual relations. In fact, it is neither the bodily transformations nor the sexual excitation experienced at puberty that serve to elaborate the difference between the male and female sexes at the level of the psychical apparatus.

What do expressions such as "to be a couple" or "to make a couple" suggest? Can they be understood as a "space of repetition"? Or as a "space of creation"?

I suggest that the initial encounter and subsequent task of maintaining a relationship between a man and a woman, on the erotic as much as on the emotional level, is a true psychic creation. And, further, that this requires the constant pressure of the sexual drive, as defined by Freud, to gain access to, and flourish in, both the ideational life of the couple and their love life.

Sexual desire and love

Falling in love, at whatever age, is a typically adolescent operation. The romantic encounter involves the enactment of two fantasy scenarios, through the autosuggestion of each of the protagonists, or through the effects of suggestion of one of them on the other, in relation to infantile prototypes. Love, as Freud noted, always makes the lover very receptive to suggestion. Hence, love at first sight! In the words of André Breton (1987/1937), love is when you meet someone who "gives you some news about yourself" (p. 9).

DOI: 10.4324/9781003471042-5

In adolescence, the relationship most often begins with a desire to merge with another person, from whom it will often be difficult to disentangle oneself without too much harm. There is quest to rediscover body-to-body, flesh-to-flesh contact with the primordial mother, fusional sensuality with the object of primary excitation/satisfaction, paradise lost. But the love-object is no longer maternal, it is the body of another person, a stranger. It is a question of leaving one's familiar space and moving towards the stranger, towards the unknown that is as strange as it is disturbing, yet so attractive! Adolescence is a period of transition, a process of separation.

Once the flare-up of love at first sight and the irresistible attraction of bodies, which contribute to the illusion of merging into one, have passed, sexual desire inevitably becomes more disjointed due to the difference between the sexes. It exposes each person to the risk posed by the other, who is a radical stranger.

A boy looks to his female partner for sexual pleasure and, above all, phallic reassurance. Castration anxiety requires it! He may give love in exchange for this conquest. A girl, however, expects a boy to love her and may give her body in exchange for love. Both of them will often very quickly see that this has its limits.

Male desire, generally speaking, is conquering, and the man's penis is visible and erectile. Its relation to the other sex is what gives rise to attraction and fascination, desire, fright and excitation.

While the penis can be brandished at will as a sign of power, its external nature nonetheless makes it fragile, and the sign risks becoming one of powerlessness; for it is the quintessentially irreducible sign of the powerlessness of man's ego to control what is the most important thing for him: the erection of his virile power. This is the domain where the unconscious asserts itself in the most untimely way. Hence, perhaps, the extraordinary valorization, not to say divinization, of the phallus in majesty. Jean Laplanche said, not without humour: "The fiasco is man's honour," for animals (*les bêtes*) do not experience this, they copulate "stupidly" (*bêtement*).

Male desire, rooted in the ability to symbolize the part for the whole, is tempted by fetishism, by separating off the desirable parts of a woman's body from the whole: breasts, neck, curves, legs, or "You've got beautiful eyes, you know!" Women know how to use this as bait.

Female desire is more interiorized and less portrayable; like her genitals, it is unrepresentable. A woman refers to her interiority, even if this is only revealed to her through exchanges of glances and in the union of bodies.

The feminine sphere can in fact be represented in two very different ways, either from the angle of the phallic/castrated opposition of the phallic organization, which harks back to castration anxiety, or from the angle of the opening and closing of the body, which harks back to intrusion and penetration anxieties, which I call "anxieties related to the feminine sphere" in both sexes.

A woman cannot give herself fully without love. "Love is the story of women's lives; it is an episode in the lives of men," wrote Madame de Staël in 1796.

The sexual relationship

The enactment of fantasies is a way of binding the libido, which facilitates the emergence of desire and maintains it during the unbinding of ecstatic pleasure. The communication of fantasy scenarios, prior to lovemaking, is part of seduction. During the act of love, this communication is more difficult, because it involves revealing, sharing or erotically imposing fantasies that are often incestuous or masochistic, thereby contributing to ecstatic pleasure. It is an erotic game. No fantasy is perverse; what is perverse is the domination and manipulation that is exerted over someone. After lovemaking, it is less common for lovers to continue to talk about love. And yet, in parallel with tenderness, the enactment of new affect-laden representations can maintain the libidinal pole of the constant pressure, as well as desire. But this is an art that no longer has currency in our civilization of "fast-food" and "fast-love." Up to this point, I have only been discussing the so-called "perverse" polymorphous component, which is normal and desirable, of all human psychosexuality.

Today, what Freud called "civilized sexual morality" is no longer what it used s be! Ecstatic sexual pleasure has become a right, and a demand. This does nothing to reassure men's castration anxiety, particularly if their phallic cathexis, feminine identification and paternal support are not very secure. And in women, it can even be said that the pursuit of an orgasm at any price has simply developed envy of the penis/phallus that is resistant to any desire for the libidinal penis.

Impotence and frigidity have by no means disappeared as a result of social change. Although sexual liberation has given women the power to consciously separate their erotic desire from their desire to procreate, it has not favoured their access to the feminine dimension, nor has it made men feel that they still have a major role to play in it.

We are too inclined to denounce the evolution of morals for having given women more autonomy and even power and deprived men of their virile privileges. Should we not stigmatize a certain frigidity and impotence, in both sexes, and prepare ourselves for the psychic work required by an encounter and the task of maintaining an erotic relationship?

Although in the social, political and economic spheres, the fight for equality between the sexes is essential and must be waged constantly, in the sexual sphere it is harmful if it tends to be confused with the abolition of the difference between the sexes, which must be exalted on account of the antagonism between the libido and the ego's defences.

The dissymmetry of the difference between the sexes is enriched by identifications. A man will also feel dominated by a woman's capacity for submission, receptivity and penetration. The more a man can defeat a woman, the more powerful he is. The more sexually submissive a woman is, the more power she has over her lover. A woman's defeat is a woman's power. It is in this sexual relationship of ecstatic pleasure that the feminine component of a woman is created in its most accomplished form, as well as the masculine component of a man.

Antagonistic to phallic logic and driven by castration anxiety, which exists only to deny, dominate, destroy or shun the feminine sphere, the masculine/feminine pairing is built through a co-creation and through discovering the female genitalia. This is what I have called the "work of the feminine," in both sexes.

Encountering and maintaining an erotic loving relationship between a man and a woman is a constant process, one that has to be reworked over and over again. This is because the feminine sphere is in a constant state of elaborating and de-elaborating the refusal to acknowledge the feminine component that lies dormant in each of us. The feminine dimension must therefore always be reconquered by both men and women. It is what sustains desire.

In my opinion, this is the pre-condition for a true emancipation that avoids the war between the sexes and the domination of one by the other. It is then that men have the possibility of no longer being afraid of women (Cournut, 2001).

The lover-for-ecstatic-pleasure

The promise of the Oedipal father that a girl has fantasized about can only be rediscovered and fulfilled in adulthood by a "lover-for-ecstatic pleasure."

It will therefore be necessary to wait, as a woman will wait, for a "lover-for-ecstatic pleasure" to reveal her genital feminine dimension. This will truly be an experience of sexual differentiation, a co-creation of the feminine and the masculine dimensions.

A lover, provided that his ego can also submit to the constant libidinal pressure, will carry it into the woman's body, opening up and sometimes revealing her "feminine dimension." This implies that he is also able to relinquish control of his ego for a time, and abandon his anal and phallic defences, to overcome fantasies of a penis that tends above all to verify its solidity in the sexual relationship, and not to be terrorized by fantasies linked to the danger of the body of the woman/mother. It also implies that his fear of his own archaic mother, of his own ecstatic pleasure or of that of the woman does not lead him only to discharge or to a return to the ego.

Pleasure and orgasm remain in the service of binding, of returning to the ego, whereas ecstatic pleasure is unbinding, an experience outside the ego entailing a loss of limits, going beyond the ego's pleasure principle. It is then that the lover will be able to confront the conflict in a woman between her libido and the resistance of her ego.

In spite of her resistance, the breach created by the constant pressure of the libido proves easier for the sexual organ of a woman, whose destiny it is to be open. This is why access to her genitality is both easier, because she is helped by the man, but more problematic than a man's, because she has to meet the man who can give her ecstatic pleasure.

What does a woman want? *Che vuoi?* A woman wants two contradictory things. Her ego abhors defeat, but her sexual organ wants it, and furthermore, demands it. She wants her own downfall, the man's "masculine dimension," insofar as it is antagonistic to the "phallic dimension" – the infantile sexual theory that exists only to avoid the difference between the sexes, and therefore her "feminine sphere." It wants vast quantities of libido and erotic masochism. This is the scandal of the feminine sphere. A woman's "work of the feminine" lies in surpassing this constitutive conflict, whether she denies it or not, of female sexuality; however, this work has to be carried out over and over again.

I contend that everything that the ego and superego find intolerable contributes precisely to ecstatic pleasure. In other words, the act of forcing one's way in, the misuse of power, the loss of control, the erasure of limits, possession, in short, "defeat," with all its polysemous meanings.

This supposes, however, that the ego of a woman, like that of a man, is able to agree to let go of its anal and phallic defences in the face of genitality. And, further, that these defences, which can justifiably be called a "repudiation of the feminine sphere," are not governed by fear, contempt or hatred of the feminine sphere, which can lead to destructive violence.

The lover-for-ecstatic pleasure also acts as a separating third party to wrest the woman from her archaic relationship with her mother: if the mother did not give the girl a penis, she did not give her a vagina either. It is by revealing her vagina to her as a whole sexual organ, through ecstatic sexual pleasure, that a lover can wrest a woman from her autoerotic relationship and from her pregenital mother.

It is thus a question of a twofold change of object, from the pregenital mother to the Oedipal father, that is to say to the genital mother, and from the Oedipal father to the lover-for-ecstatic pleasure. The change of object is a change of submission: from anal submission to the mother, which the daughter tried to evade through penis-envy, to abandoned libidinal submission with desire and pleasure to the lover. Since the dawn of time, men have had to drag girls away from the night of women, from the "queens of the night."

A woman submits out of love. She cannot give herself fully without love.

It is never simple to let oneself be defeated by the other. The feminine sphere always has to be reconquered by the masculine sphere. This is also what maintains the requirement of desire to accept what is extraneous, disturbing and familiar, provided that the danger of penetration is not confused with a danger of pregenital intrusion.

Making herself the object of the other, of the lover, implies that the woman is not dispossessed of her status as a subject. It is about abandoning herself to the other, losing herself, but without being desubjectivized, while still being able to rediscover herself. "Belonging to the other" (Pickman, 2016) is a fine expression which harks back to the notion of the "reflexive middle voice" theorized by Freud (1915), that of the double reversal (i.e. turning round upon the subject's own self and reversal into its opposite) in *Instincts and their Vicissitudes.* As Freud writes, "An extraneous person is once more sought as object; this person, in consequence of the alteration which has taken place in the instinctual aim, has to take over the role of the subject" (p. 127).

The term "new subject" is used by Freud to refer to an active drive agent, an external protagonist capable of satisfying the demand for passive satisfaction of the self. It is the reversal of the instinctual drive aim into the passive mode which calls for the emergence of an external subject through whom the self can satisfy itself.

If there is a place where the entry of the constant pressure into the ego can be perceived, unfolded and experienced in an enriching way, it is in the relationship of sexual ecstasy. The co-creation of the adult feminine and masculine components and sexual ecstasy are part of those mutative experiences which bring about a reorganization of the psychical economy, and enrich the ego with affect-laden representations.

The adult libidinal "genital" sphere is what is most difficult and most violent, and what mobilizes most strongly the anal, faecal and phallic defences that can be called the "refusal of the feminine sphere." It requires an integrative effort on the part of the ego in the face of the constant pressure of the libido in sexuality, and it is the violence of this ordeal that can stand up to and oppose the violence of the regressive ascendancy of the archaic mother, and the violence attributed to the death drive, both of which pull towards non-differentiation.

What is deeply terrifying, for both sexes, is the proximity of the mother's sexual organ from which they came. This is the object of the taboo, of the repressed par excellence. This greed of the instinctual drive pressure, which is always unsatisfied, cannot fail to be terrifying if it harks back to fears of being eaten up and absorbed into the mother's body, an object of terror as well as the paradise lost of fusion/confusion. Both men and women will always be faced with the terror of the archaic mother, with phallic defences and reciprocal envious impulses. Homosexual pregenital fixations are difficult to overcome.

Yet it is by confronting and overcoming these terrors that sexual ecstasy is created. Freud (1912) had the audacity to claim that "anyone who is to be really free and happy in love must have surmounted his respect for women and have come to terms with the idea of incest with his mother or sister" (p. 187).

These are only ideas, but they imply that ecstatic sexual pleasure comes very close to the incestuous core of the unconscious.

No event in the life of an adult can be compared to a relationship of ecstatic sexual pleasure, which is one of the most powerful ways of putting humans in direct contact with the deepest layers of mental life where primary processes reign supreme, and also of exalting the antagonisms that are constitutive of the mind and erotic masochism (Zaltzman, 1976).

Female homosexuality

Male homosexuality, governed by castration anxiety, may manifest itself as a quest for the penis, at the erotic level, but also, at the symbolic phallic level, as a quest to be a penis-bearer. This is often due to an absence of or insufficient phallic transmission by the father.

Female homosexuality has as its crucible the "night of the mothers" the shadow of the maternal sphere (Schaeffer, 2015). Could the "dark continent" of women be maternal in origin?

Primary homosexuality is the prelude to this. It takes into account an erotic cathexis of the mother, of the seductive mother and the first loving exchanges between mother and infant, and seals the original maternal feminine imprint in both sexes. As a deferred effect, it provides the fantasy of a lost paradise.

However, if it persists and hinders the differentiation of parental *imagos*, the attraction of this homosexual imprint will remain predominant and defensively split-off, threatening to contaminate, with its hallucinatory potential, any subsequent relationship in both sexes with femininity and the feminine sphere. Marguerite Duras (1967/1964) describes it in terms of "rapture."

It seems, however, that this homosexuality remains more incestuous between mother and daughter. The identical nature of their genitalia requires a strong anti-cathexis to subject the erogeneity of the little girl's sexual organs to primary repression.

If primal repression did not occur under optimal conditions, if the mother was too seductive, either through her maternal care or through the ascendancy she exerted over the daughter's body and mind, these incestuous seductive behaviours may compromise the change of object and the future woman's capacity for ecstatic pleasure. Mother-daughter incest has been considered the fundamental homosexual fantasy, and regression to primary homosexuality in the treatment represents shared erotic completeness.

How can the girl free herself from this ascendancy of the wild maternal sphere when the intensity of the libidinal impulses of the fixation to the pre-Oedipal mother is "incommensurable," according to Freud, i.e. entailing vast quantities of energy?

For the girl, the shadow of maternal incest remains a threat that can only be removed by turning towards the father in the Oedipal stage. If the change of object did not take place, hatred may remain – hatred of the mother, hatred of herself, hatred that is mixed up with unconscious hatred of the mother.

The female homosexual relationship denies the function and value of the penis by revealing the vagina and female ecstatic pleasure. The radical split between signs of virility and femininity indicates an anti-cathexis of psychic bisexuality, as an integration of the capacities for Oedipal identification with the two protagonists of the primal scene, and thus of the difference between the sexes. There is therefore a double split: between the erotic feminine sphere and the maternal feminine sphere, and between the masculine and feminine spheres.

Acted-out homosexuality, in certain cases, can amount to a reappropriation of wounded or lost femininity.

At the onset of menopause, some women who had previously experienced love and desire with a man find themselves in love with a woman, often a younger woman. In this way, they retain their femininity, their feminine identity, vicariously. They see a reflection of themselves in the young woman they love, a double of what they imagine themselves to have been in their youth (Schaeffer, 2005). This is most often a female homosexuality that does not involve sex or genitality, where the current of tenderness and love predominates.

Female narcissism

The erotic encounter that involves love puts the body to the test of the other, with risks for the ego and narcissism. What is the nature of the links between the body and narcissism? What does narcissism owe to the body?

The most archaic traces of ecstatic pleasure are registered in the flesh of autoeroticism and primary narcissism. This primary narcissism is nonetheless underpinned by an attachment of "maternal preoccupation," including both the care and seduction of the primary object, nourished by parental narcissistic projection which makes the infant *His Majesty the Baby.*

The experience of the "mirror stage," according to Jacques Lacan (2006/1949), seems to throw light on the constitution of primary narcissism in both men and women. The infant looks into his mother's eyes as she looks at him, confirming what he sees in the mirror. It is a moment of recognition by the object of the specular image. Secondary narcissism is caught up in a relationship with the other, where the cathexis of the object of love returns to the ego, whereas primary narcissism refers only to the subject's own body.

While men's narcissism is primarily phallic, due to castration anxiety about their penis, women's narcissism is more bodily, even if it can also be cathected in a phallic mode. Their whole body is involved, but it is subject to the reassurance of the gaze of the other, which makes women dependent on the gaze, desire and love of the object.

The need for recognition in phallic narcissism is a need to be admired, whereas in female narcissism it is a need to be desired. A woman whose narcissism cannot be based on phallic valorization remains more dependent on the object that confirms her narcissistic image, and she constructs her libidinal object on the desire to be desired. But if she is dependent only on her mirror image, if she has not built up sufficiently gratifying internal objects, and if a loving object does not give her, through the brilliance of its gaze, another mirror, she runs the risk of a depressive collapse at whenever she is faced with separation.

In the event of a break-up, betrayal or bereavement, what is suddenly missing is this gaze, and the woman can then lose her symbolic bearings, as if she were nothing.

Instinctual drive violence

It is important to note that the force of the drives is attributed solely to those that involve destructiveness. Rapists, sex murderers or paedophiles are said to have been driven by their powerful "impulses." According to psychoanalysts these impulses have their source in the id. But should we deny that they can nonetheless be enriching for the mind? Why is it that we find it so difficult to take into account the irruptive dimension of the sexual drives as well as their nourishing dimension?

Violence is not just on the side of hatred, perversion or destruction. An erotic relationship requires – due to the fusion of the drives – just as much violence, and even cruelty, as desire or tenderness. Eradicating the dimension of aggression and transgression from the sexual act has harmful and sometimes catastrophic consequences for sexuality. A loss of desire, increasing recourse to regressive and addictive forms of sexuality, and anxiety about impotence are widely observable today. In my clinical practice I frequently come across people suffering from a lack of interest in sex, vaginismus, or who have no sexual relations at all.

Sexual desire is always violent, both for the person who feels it and for the person who is the object of this desire.

Feminine erotic masochism

But why is there instinctual drive violence? I would venture to say that it is because the scandal of the feminine sphere is erotic masochism. It is no coincidence that Freud links the "enigma of the feminine" with another enigma in the form of "mysterious masochistic tendencies." And I would even go as far as to say that in order to become a woman it is necessary to combine the scandal of the feminine sphere with another scandal, that of masochism.

It is this movement of reversal from activity to active passivity, that of the feminine masochistic movement, described by Catherine Parat (1959), that specifies the feminine Oedipus.

Personally, I speak of feminine erotic masochism, rather than erotogenic masochism. For Freud, in 1924, this erotogenic masochism was primary; he saw it as a fixation point (and nucleus of the first operation of binding) which remains in the organism where it is bound by libidinal sympathetic excitation (1924, p. 163). He saw it as a vital defence against destructiveness. For Benno Rosenberg (1991), this operation of binding is confused with primary drive fusion which, as such, he points out, is masochistic in essence. Mental life depends on this first operation of binding. If it does not exist, or is defective, neither deferred satisfaction nor displacement can take place, and the drive can only deteriorate into excitation, fulfilling its aim either through discharge, immediate or violent acting out, self-destructive or hetero-destructive, or through self-destructive psychosomatic discharge.

As for "feminine masochism," according to Freud, in men it consists in eroticizing the pain and humiliation suffered by women. It is a masturbatory version with a fetishist turn.

Feminine erotic masochism is of a completely different nature; it is constitutive of a feminine sphere beyond the phallic dimension, and contributes to an erotic relationship between the feminine and masculine spheres.

As I understand it, it is psychical and not perverse or acted-out. It is a capacity for openness and abandonment to strong libidinal quantities and to possession by the sexual object. When unbinding occurs, paradoxically it provides the binding necessary for the cohesion of the ego so that the latter can unravel, and it requires a reliable object. We can then speak of "non-dangerous de-liaisons."[1]

Masochism, the "guardian of secrecy," according to Karl Abraham, helps to shape the inside, interiority, returning to oneself. It is an indispensable auxiliary for analytic treatment. It is the inventor of guilt, in the secrecy of its greatest pleasure. The phallic dimension cathects the visible and the exterior, while masochism cathects the interior and interiorization. According to Benno Rosenberg, masochism, the "guardian of life," is perhaps the guarantor of ecstatic pleasure, but could it also be the guarantor of feminine narcissism?

As early as 1919, Freud addressed the erotic Oedipal character of a girl's masochistic desire in his article "A child is being beaten" (Freud, 1919), which he discussed at length. It is her guilt for this Oedipal desire that leads the girl to express it, in regressive mode, in the second particularly repressed stage of the fantasy: "Daddy, beat me! Daddy, rape me!"

Anna, Freud's daughter, in a lecture given in 1922 (Anna Freud, 1922), confirmed the Oedipal nature of the masochistic fantasy in girls. Echoing her own experience on her father's couch, she suggests that a young female patient was struggling against fantasies, whose erotic nature she was aware of as well as their connection with the girl's love for her father.

But Freud soon returned to his phallic theory. In 1925, he said that in little girls it is the clitoris that is being beaten (Freud, 1925). Having his daughter Anna on his couch, with her beating fantasies, did not make things any easier!

I would distance myself, therefore, from the view according to which feminine is equated with "castrated" or "infantile," and argue instead for a feminine erotic masochism that is genital and contributes to a sexual relationship in which ecstatic pleasure is shared between a man and a woman.

The woman's ego can then appropriate the experience of having sexual ecstasy wrested from her.

"There is a sort of glory of subjection in women," writes Marguerite Duras,

> but many women deny it. It is the reign of subjection. I regret that many women are unaware of all of this... I believe that without it, sexuality in women is weak and incomplete. It is as if they carried within themselves their own Middle Ages, as if they carried within themselves their own primary barbarity intact, that had been covered in sand over time, for centuries
>
> (Duras & Ceton, 2012, p. 83)

What does a woman want? She wants both to be wanted and loved, which is not always differentiated in women. A woman cannot give herself fully without love. This is what makes her dependent and submissive to the domination of men in sexual relations. This means she is more threatened by the loss of the sexual object than by the loss of a sexual organ. The Oedipal sexuality of boys and the "compromised" sexuality of adult men are more easily structured around anxiety related to the loss of the sexual organ.

Opera acknowledges this dissymmetry.

"I'll kill you if you leave me!", Don José tells Carmen.

And Madame Butterfly says: "I'll kill myself if you leave me!"

This erotic masochism makes a woman in love say to her lover: "Take me wherever you want to go, I belong to you, possess me, conquer me!" Her abandonment calls for the security of a reliable and loving lover. The real aim of masochism is sexual ecstasy.

The lover, provided that his ego has also been able to submit to the constant libidinal pressure, will carry it into the woman's body. He will have to confront in her the conflict between her libido and the resistance of her ego. "Woman's essence is a devotedness that manifests itself as resistance," writes Kierkegaard (1958, p. 121).

The lover is to a woman's sexuality what the drive is to the ego: the need to accept what is extraneous, which is both disturbing and familiar. Women are thus, in spite of themselves, obliged to carry out "work on the feminine sphere." No woman can allow herself to be penetrated unless she has succeeded in transforming her pregenital intrusion anxieties into "anxieties related to the feminine sphere," into genital penetration anxieties. The fantasy of being raped, which is highly eroticized and a frequent occurrence in adolescence, often marks the transition from one form of anxiety to the other. The feminine sphere – that of the difference between the sexes – is thus what the lover wrests from a woman by destroying her repudiation of the feminine sphere.

Sexual ecstasy is part of the rediscovery of this moment of the "defeat" of infantile narcissism violated by erotic impulses, a foundational moment of sexual desire created by primary identification with the mother who has become a lover again, during the phase of the "censorship of the woman-as-lover." Thus it reproduces the inevitable association between eroticism and masochism.

I have chosen to draw on Freud's "metapsychological witch" to define the "feminine sphere" as the ego's capacity to admit large quantities of unbound excitation into itself, not to be traumatically breached by them but, on the contrary, to be nourished by them and to use them as a source of growth. This is what used to be called a "strong ego." In fact a strong ego, one that has integrated the feminine sphere and therefore bisexuality, is a very flexible ego, one that can expand without exposing itself to the risk of fragmenting or imploding.

Female castration anxiety

A father's recognition of his daughter's femininity is essential. It is this paternal gaze, which, according to Winnicott, is different from the mother's "mirror" gaze, that will mark the destiny of the woman's femininity in the sense of wanting to be looked at and desired by a man. It is a gaze that says "You're a pretty little girl," but also, in an non-incestuous Oedipal register, "One day your Prince will come!"

This paternal cathexis is what can prevent the depressive risk caused by feelings of not having a sexual organ, or of having a castrated sexual organ. While a woman's narcissism cannot be supported by phallic confirmation, she remains more dependent on the object that has confirmed her narcissistic image, and she constructs her libidinal object according to this desire to be desired.

Some women today who have experienced the liberation of their bodies and the mastery of procreation, know and are able to feel that their "anxieties related to the feminine sphere" cannot be assuaged or satisfactorily resolved by a realization in a "phallic" mode.

More precisely, the fact of not being desired or no longer being desired by a man takes them back to painful feelings of not having a sexual organ, or of having a sexual organ that is denied, and revives the injury they felt as little girls when they were forced to organize themselves in a phallic mode to cope with the ordeal of perceiving the difference between the sexes. This is where their "castration anxiety" lies.

I have therefore chosen to define castration anxiety in relation to sexuality, desire and erotic potency, and the threat that failure or loss represents for them. But castration anxiety also manifests itself in the face of a threat of failure or real loss concerning a realization that is highly cathected in the phallic register. This is the case for a theorization that situates female castration anxiety on the side of failures of procreation.

Note

1 This is an allusion to (1) the title of Choderlos de Laclos' 1782 novel *Les Liaisons dangereuses,* (2) J. Schaeffer's (1997) book *Le refus du féminin* (translated into English as *The Universal Refusal* (Schaeffer, 2011)), and (3) the title of Raymond Cahn's (1991) book *Adolescence et folie. Les dé-liaisons dangereuses.* In French psychoanalysis *liaison/déliaison* = binding/unbinding.

References

Breton, A. (1987/1937). *Mad Love,* trans. Anne Caws. Lincoln: University of Nebraska Press.

Cahn, R. (1991). *Adolescence et folie. Les dé-liaisons dangereuses*. Presses Universitaires de France.

Cournut, J. (2001). *Pourquoi les hommes ont peur des femmes?* Paris: Presses Universitaires de France.

Duras, M. (1967/1964). *The Rapture of L. V. Stein*. London: H. Hamilton.

Duras, M. & Ceton, J-P. (2012). *Entretiens avec Marguerite Duras, « On ne peut pas avoir écrit Lol V. Stein et désirer être encore à l'écrire*. Paris: François Bourin.

Freud, S. (1912). On the universal tendency to debasement in the sphere of love. *S.E.* 11. London: Hogarth, pp. 179–190.

Freud, S. (1915). *Instincts and their Vicissitudes. S.E. 14.* London: Hogarth, pp. 117–140.

Freud, S. (1919). A child is being beaten. *S.E.* 19. London: Hogarth, pp. 177–204.

Freud, A. (1922). Schlagephantasie und Tagtraum. *Imago*, 8: 317–332. (English translation: Beating phantasies and daydreams. *International Journal of Psychoanalysis,* 4: 89–102, 1923.)

Freud, S. (1924). The economic problem of masochism. *S.E.* 19. London: Hogarth, pp. 159–170.

Freud, S. (1925). Some psychical consequences of the anatomical distinction between the sexes. *S.E.* 19. London: Hogarth, pp. 248–258.

Kierkegaard, S. (1958/1843). *The Seducer's Diary*, trans. Hong, H.V. & Hong, E.V. Princeton: Princeton University Press, 1977.

Lacan, J. (2006/1949). The mirror stage as formative of the *I* function as revealed in psychoanalytic experience. In: Écrits, trans. B. Fink. New York, NY: Norton, pp. 75–81.

Masson, J.M. Editor (1985). *The Complete Letters of Sigmund Freud to Wilhelm Fliess,* 1887–1904. Cambridge, MA: Belknap.

Parat, C. (1959). La place du mouvement masochique dans l'évolution de la femme. *Revue française de psychanalyse,* 23(3): 305–352.

Pickmann, C.N. (2016). S'appartenir à l'Autre. Remarques sur le masochisme érogène. *La clinique lacanienne,* 28(2): 137–154.

Rosenberg, B. (1991). Masochisme mortifère et masochisme gardien de vie. In: *Monographies de la Revue française de Psychanalyse*. Paris: Presses Universitaires de France.

Schaeffer, J. (2005). Quel retour d'âge? Début de la fin ou fin du début? Les pulsions au milieu de la vie. *Revue française de psychanalyse,* 69(4): 1013–1030.

Schaeffer, J. (2015). La nuit des Mères. Ombre de l'homosexualité féminine. *Revue française de psychanalyse,* 79(3): 735–748.

Zaltzmann, N. (1976). Du sexe opposé. *Nouvelle Revue de Psychanalyse*, 14: 183–206.

Chapter 6

The feminine and maternal spheres

An inevitable antagonism

The conflict between the feminine and maternal spheres

The conflict specific to women is the inevitable antagonism that exists between three poles of their fulfilment: motherhood, their erotic sexual life, and their social fulfilment, or so-called "phallic" fulfilment. Unlike in men, these three poles are inevitably in conflict and also impose a "demand for work."

This antagonism between the feminine and the maternal spheres runs through a woman's life (Schaeffer, 2002). The split in a man, clearly identified by Freud, between the mother and the whore, has more to do with his object relationship than with his own body. In women, however, the antagonism is more between the narcissistic and object-related cathexes of the erotic feminine dimension and the bodily and psychic, passionate and tender maternal dimension. The body is at the heart of women's sexuality and narcissism.

It is important to refer to an antagonism rather than a split between the feminine and maternal spheres. To confuse them is to reproduce the eternal definition of women as bodies destined for reproduction, not as individuals animated by sexual desire, other than as unbridled seductresses. This takes us back again to Freud's idea that, in the female version of the Oedipus complex, the desire for a child, as the equivalent of the penis for girls, precedes erotic desire.

The anthropologist Françoise Héritier (1996) asserts that women beget their daughters, while men cannot beget their sons. To reproduce identically, men are dependent on women's bodies. This is what constitutes an injustice between men and women, not penis envy and castration. Women, then, have something that men do not have.

A cartoon by Claire Bretecher[1] made a feminist who had just learned from an ultrasound scan that she was pregnant with a boy say: "What I can't stand is having balls in my belly!" This joke caricatures the refusal to accept a man's penis and its domination, which has even led some feminists to refuse motherhood insofar as it is the mark of a virile presence.

As we know, the feminist movement has led to considerable progress, in particular, the ability to consciously dissociate a woman's erotic desire from

DOI: 10.4324/9781003471042-6

her desire for a child, and to give her back the power to decide on procreation. But can it be said that this has contributed to freeing women from the ascendancy of the primitive mother, and to gaining access to the feminine sphere in sexual relations?

Experience and clinical evidence bear witness to the existence and destiny of a twofold current: the erotic feminine sphere and the maternal sphere. The two do not necessarily go well together. From the time of being a baby girl until the menopause, what plays out in a woman is an antagonism and alternation between erotic and maternal cathexes. This takes place in the little girl, first with her mother, then later on in the woman once she has become a mother, in connection with what has been described concerning the "censorship of the woman-as-lover" (Braunschweig & Fain, 1975).

It is a woman's destiny to be torn between her social, or so-called "phallic" fulfilment, her erotic life and her life as a mother. It requires psychical work to reconcile these antagonisms so that being penetrated, receiving the penis for ecstatic pleasure, does not conflict too strongly with keeping, nourishing and helping a child to grow inside her; and so that all these pleasures in the same place are not an object of scandal.

We can only hope that once a girl becomes a woman she will be able to reconcile the erotic feminine sphere with the maternal sphere, in relation to her mother's body, so that these two feminine capacities, while remaining in tension, can be combined without splitting in her future body as a woman and mother.

A woman who gives birth: goddess or mammal?

I had the honour of discussing a clinical research paper by Alexandra Bouchard (2023), on the theme of "The feminine sphere and the challenge of childbirth." Among the antagonisms that exist in women's bodies and minds, she explored those that exist between the feminine and the maternal spheres, and between the phallic and maternal spheres. In the conclusion to her paper, she writes: "Childbirth represents a challenge for the feminine sphere, confronting it once again with the difference between the sexes and generations, and should perhaps be considered as a special time in the psychosexual development of women" (p. 242).

Could it be that the similarities between defloration and childbirth that she identifies are due to the confrontation with the sexual dimension of childbirth, or to the fact that it is the first time? Is not the essential issue the terror of blood, which Freud (1918) refers to as a taboo?

Is childbirth equated in fantasy with a sexual act?

Could the unbearable conflict be due to the fact that the child passes through the same vaginal canal as the penis, and that the sensations produced there are of a sexual nature?

For the mind, this is an absolute scandal, so much so that the Church Fathers preferred to adopt the infantile sexual theory of the child-excrement, like the *lumpf* in Little Hans (Freud, 1909), and defined childbirth as: *Inter urinas et faeces nascimur*. The vagina has no acceptable existence, according to their logic, since the mother, Mary, as well as her own mother, both gave birth by means of an immaculate conception, i.e. without a sexual act. So there is a clear split between the sexual and the maternal spheres, the excremental *versus* the mammalian, and purity *versus* the Madonna.

In every child's mind, the mother is, and must remain, a virgin. This persists in the minds of some adult men, in the form of a "split between the mother and the whore."

The confusion of zones, sensations and the intense quantity of excitation can certainly lead to childbirth being likened to an orgasm. Especially as the combination of pain and excitation may be linked to the experience of unbinding, of being outside of the ego, of ecstasy and the loss of the limits of feminine ecstatic pleasure.

The fantasy of reverse coitus is therefore possible. It can also be thought of in terms of part-objects, by a simple inversion of movement and displacement of the part for the whole, taking us back to Freudian theory.

Childbirth is the most unthinkable and transgressive act that exists. It is situated between two poles: what is most animal and what is most sacred. A woman who gives birth is both a mammal and a goddess.

Can we speak, then, of a split between the feminine and the maternal spheres? It is important to emphasize the psychic, dynamic value of repression: unlike splitting, which breaks the links between what is split-off and awareness, repression allows for alternation. This makes it possible to speak of an antagonism between the feminine and the maternal spheres, the prelude to which is the "censorship of woman-as-lover."

Does a fantasized Oedipal or incestuous fulfilment exist?

The child and the penis use the same passage, but in reverse directions. The interpenetration of bodies and physiological and psychic regression on a formal level are favourable to the production of incestuous fantasy scenarios. What might the objects of these scenarios of incestuous fulfilment be?

The father?

Is the child the fulfilment of the paternal promise of the gift of a child as a substitute for the penis (Bouchard, 2023)? Or is there a risk, during childbirth, of enacting representations of an incestuous fulfilment with the father, the transgression of the prohibition of incest being acted out in his body (Bydlowski, 2000)?

The Oedipal complex has an anti-incestuous function. Once the Oedipal organization has been established, the incestuous fantasy is blocked by the superego, an agency that operates a repression as soon as an incestuous threat arises. The risk of transgression lies in fact in a failure of the superego function. Or could these representations be a scenario for elaborating the incestuous fantasy?

The mother?

The woman giving birth was indeed the one who penetrated her mother backwards. It is this body-to-body contact, this excess of intimacy, rather than childbirth itself, that carries the risk of incest, and what is most unbearable is that a daughter may have provoked erotic impulses in her mother.

My hypothesis is that the daughter is subjected not only to fantasies, but also to experiences of incorporation. The mother/daughter relationship is a body-to-body relationship, and can be reciprocal. We know that some mothers, when their daughters give birth, experience a surge of milk, and what used to be called "trenches."

It is because of this experience of incorporation, in my opinion, that violence and aggression can be unleashed. The girl's vagina must remain in the shadow of the maternal sphere, protected from the primary repression of the vagina. This is what allows the taboo of "primordial incest" (Cabrol, 2011) to be repressed.

What is unrepresentable, in both sexes, is the proximity of the mother's sexual organ through which they were born. The primary repression of the vagina concerns both the maternal vagina and the girl's. The lifting of this repression can be traumatic, when a daughter is involved too directly with her mother's sexuality, and especially with one of her mother's lovers. The fantasy is one of a vagina for two, and the daughter is prevented from appropriating her own.

The child?

The baby has the impudence to penetrate its mother backwards, giving her extraordinary sensations.

Later on, we know the extent to which a baby can become an "erotic toy" for its mother, as Freud wrote. It is important that the mother's erotic dimension is protected by repression, so that the baby does not become a phobic object for a phobic mother.

After a mother has carried the body of an infant inside her own body and shaped it with her own flesh, and even more so if she gives it her breast, sexual impulses can be transmitted from body to body, from flesh to flesh. It is "the flesh of her flesh."

The infant at the breast is an insatiable cannibal, whose "excited love is cupboard love" (Winnicott, 1947, p. 201). Melanie Klein tells the story of a small child who pointed to his mother's breast as she was feeding his little brother, and asked: "Mummy, is that what you used to bite me with?"

Is not the shared fantasy one of devouring each other? The baby, who for the mother was still only a part of herself, a part-object, elicits her infantile sexual theories. Was this infant who fed on her flesh not also devoured by its mother, since it was a guest in her womb? Who devoured whom? The ogre and ogress of fairy tales answer this question: the belly of the wolf who ate the child is opened up and pebbles are put inside. Very few studies explore the cannibalistic impulses of the mother ("she-wolf and bitch" according to Marguerite Duras). The orgy of breast-feeding is a shared feast.

The erotic breast and the maternal breast, evoking both hunger and love, are both just waiting to be bitten, sucked, chewed, kneaded and devoured. But a taboo separates them: the primary taboo of incest and the taboo of cannibalism. These are the two fundamental anthropological taboos.

Repression is often required when, during breast-feeding, the voracity of the little ogre's mouth at the breast provokes uterine contractions in the mother. It is important for the mother to be able to keep repressed ecstatic pleasures unknown to herself, in the sense of the sacred horror of primeval incest, which always takes place with the primitive mother. Maternal incest is the fundamental homosexual fantasy.

This is what requires the anti-cathexis of the "censorship of the woman-as-lover" (Braunschweig & Fain, 1975), the alternation of the post-Oedipal baby of daytime reality with the hallucinatory, pregenital or Oedipal nighttime baby.

Bouchard has suggested that childbirth may be a mark of overcoming the Oedipal situation for a woman. One of the ways in which the girl's Oedipus complex is resolved, which Freud described as a long process of liberation from the mother that is sometimes never achieved, could be through the experience of childbirth.

Note

1 A French humoristic cartoonist and illustrator (b.1940–d.2020).

References

Bouchard, C. (2023). *Césariennes sur demandes maternelles. Le féminin à l'épreuve de l'accouchement,* postface de Jacqueline Schaeffer. Paris: Eres.

Braunschweig, M., & Fain, M. (1975). *La nuit, le jour. Essai psychanalytique sur le fonctionnement mental.* Paris: Presses Universitaires de France.

Bydlowski, M. (2000). *Je rêve un enfant. L'expérience intérieure de la maternité.* Paris: Odile Jacob.

Cabrol, G. (2011). Le refoulement de l'inceste primordiale. *Bulletin de la Société Psychanalytique de Paris*, 99(5): 99–103.
Freud, S. (1909). Analysis of a phobia in a five-year-old boy. *S.E.* 10. London: Hogarth, pp. 5–149.
Freud, S. (1918 [1917]). The taboo of virginity (contributions to the psychology of love, III). *S.E.* 11. London: Hogarth, pp. 193–208.
Héritier, F. (1996). *Masculin/féminin, la pensée de la différence*. Paris: Odile Jacob.
Schaeffer, J. (2002). Le parcours des antagonismes entre féminin et maternel. In: *La parentalité. Défi pour le troisième millénaire*. Paris: Presses Universitaires de France, pp. 139–155.
Winnicott, D.W. (1947). Hate in the countertransference. In: *Through Paediatrics to Psychoanalysis, Collected Papers*. London: Tavistock, 1958, pp. 194–203.

Chapter 7

The feminine sphere, the maternal sphere and the father/lover

The maternal body

The antagonism between the father and the lover

The woman's body, but particularly her flesh, is erotically stimulated by both her lover and her baby. The father/lover has a relationship with the inside of his wife's body, he plunges into her flesh. With the baby, he only comes into contact with its body, not its flesh. The infant will always remain an external object. However, his phallic organization and his castration anxiety will push him to resume his place as lover with the mother. This can sometimes prove conflictual, both for him and for the couple. It is thus the object, between the woman/mother and the woman/lover that will have to undergo a transformation.

On the mother's side, the "censorship of the woman-as-lover," which presides over the sleep/dream system, whose alternation is represented by night and day, is desexualizing for the child and resexualizing for the lover.

The father certainly manifests his own desire, but he is designated as a lover through the mother's erotic desire. It is because the mother makes herself desiring and desirable that she can transmit to the child, through censorship, the preform of the representation of a third object, another object of her desire. This proto-object can be hallucinated, because the infant can feel and fantasize that the abandonment it suffers does not mean that it is a bad object, an object of phobia, hatred or disgust, but rather that there is another object that is desired by the mother. This enables the infant to have access to the sleep/dream system too, and to create its first psychical operations, namely, hallucinatory satisfaction and its first auto-erotic experiences.

There would only be a real split if the father were excluded, and if the mother, seduced by her baby, which is at once a "sexual bomb… pleasure-seeking and constantly provocative" (Parat, 2011), used him exclusively as a "substitute for a complete sexual object" (Freud, 1905, p. 223). This would be evidence in her of a defensive struggle against feelings of anxiety or of being wounded, manifested by "sticking."

DOI: 10.4324/9781003471042-7

The "censorship of the woman-as-lover," on the contrary, permits the libidinal development and blossoming not only of the child but also of the mother, who can alternate between sexual relations and maternal care, with a full reawakening of her infantile sexuality, without the weight of the guilt of betrayal and without any blurring of her erotic sensations.

What about the lover? What is the nature of the antagonism between the father and the lover? When he is present, the father plays a decisive role in the metamorphosis of the mother/ lover. Hélène Parat (2011) rightly speaks of the protection that the father/lover must lavish on the mother in order to "limit maternal madness … temper the wild maternal dimension in her" (Abensour, 2010) and the temptation she has to let herself "slip back into pregenital delights" (Parat, 2011).

Of course, we can only concur with this mission of a father/lover. It brings into play the necessary symbolic paternal function that enables the father to separate the child from its mother and to introduce it to the social world.

But does this constitute "censorship"? I would argue that it is more a question of repression in the face of the erotic body of the woman/mother. Indeed, if this repression is not sufficiently operative, the man makes love with a "mother," and this confronts him with a primordial incestuous fantasy, which often leads to symptoms of sexual impotence.

A conflict between the maternal breast and the erotic breast

If both are treated as part-objects, the erotic breast and the maternal breast may come into conflict, and find themselves subject to a logic of repression.

A lack of repression acted out at the level of the confusion between a nourishing breast and an erotic breast can even result in impeding the right use of the censorship of the woman-as-lover. Here is an example. The husband of a patient who had recently given birth resumed sexual relations with her and, under the pretext of eroticism, started sucking and drinking the milk from her breasts. Although the patient loves her husband, she suddenly felt submerged with hatred.

The censorship of the woman-as-lover can no longer operate vis-a-vis her baby. The husband becomes in fantasy an incestuous child, in rivalry with her infant at the breast. Night and day are dreadfully intertwined.

Crossing the barrier of repression between the nourishing breast and the erotic breast gives rise to incestuous fantasies, but also, in an adult, to polymorphous perverse behaviour, like that of an infant. To continue breastfeeding her baby in peace, the patient refuses to have any sexual contact with her husband, taking charge herself of the repression in her husband's place.

A conflict between the maternal breast and the phallic penis

When the nourishing breast is treated as a part-object, it can also come into conflict with the man's phallicized penis. A father may experience feelings of envious rivalry with the baby his wife is breastfeeding, as well as with her. His phallic organization may be endangered, and his castration anxiety exacerbated.

A patient, whose wife has just given birth, finds himself relegated to the child's bedroom. His virility is threatened, and he feels powerless like a child excluded from the primal scene represented by his wife on her honeymoon with her baby, and from the primal scene that the birth of his brother in his mother's bed represented for him. His castration anxiety finds an outlet in a dream of a huge ejaculation, which he humorously associates with the fantasy that he could have painted my stairwell, which has no a lift and has just been repainted. The prowess of this penis/phallus attempts to measure itself against the enormous power of a nursing mother.

When psychic bisexuality is not confused with omnipotence and narcissistic completeness, or with the illusion of symmetry, it can be used to help work through the difference between the sexes. This work enabled the patient to rediscover his wife's feminine sphere, and they went on a honeymoon… with the baby.

References

Abensour, L. (2010). L'ombre du maternel. *Revue française de psychanalyse,* 75(5): 1297–1335.

Freud, S. (1905). Three essays on the theory of sexuality. *S.E.* 7. London: Hogarth, pp.130–243.

Parat, C. (2011). L'érotique maternel et l'interdit primaire de l'inceste. *Revue française de psychanalyse,* 75(5): 1609–1614.

Chapter 8

Feminine suffering

> I live, I die, I flare up & I drown.
> Taking pleasure in each twinge of pain.
> Then convinced my bliss cannot be denied
> And I'm about to climb joy's highest peak,
> He reminds me of all my former grief.
>
> Louise Labé (2014), Sonnet VIII (1524–1566).

I will confine myself to just a few examples of feminine suffering, and the ways in which they manifest themselves.

This suffering cannot be linked to feminine erotic masochism. However, some of them can be used by repetition compulsion to feed the moral masochism often observed in some women.

The loss of love

Freud contrasts castration anxiety in men and separation anxiety, loss of the object and love in women. He argues that the absence of castration anxiety in girls exposes them to anxieties about losing everything, which is more a loss of being than of having (Schaeffer, 2013).

A woman's dependence on love makes her more vulnerable to the loss of a sexual object than to the loss of a sexual organ, an anxiety around which the Oedipal sexuality of boys and the sexuality of male adults are more easily structured. This is why, as Freud says, she is more exposed to the loss of love, to disappointment, and finds herself so threatened by depression in the event of losing a love object.

Very often, the loss of a love object can mean losing everything, being cast back into nothingness, an experience of no longer being worth anything. In this case, the loss of an object is confused with a total narcissistic loss.

Opera clearly acknowledges this dissymmetry of the feminine or masculine position when faced with abandonment.

"I'll kill you if you leave me!", Don José tells Carmen.

And Madame Butterfly says: "I'll kill myself if you leave me!"

DOI: 10.4324/9781003471042-8

The abandoned man kills the object, in general in fantasy, whereas the abandoned woman becomes a lost object.

The loss of a loving relationship and the feelings of failure that accompany it reawaken the traces of the Oedipal failure. And the mourning of Oedipal desire has to be resumed. The devaluation caused by the loss of object-love, experienced as a narcissistic trauma, can disorganize the feminine system of self-worth, and in men it can reactivate the whole issue of castration.

The disappearance, erasure or wear and tear of the love felt for an object is an ordeal. The withdrawal of cathexis leaves a void, and the woman loses a support, an opportunity for expectation, fantasying, exaltation, excitation and self-excitation.

Suffering is an internal object that can sometimes be precious and exciting, and the lamentations of women can also be a source of enjoyment. This brings us back to the link with feminine erotic masochism.

"How I wish that I had never seen you" writes the Portuguese nun, who immediately exclaims: "I had far rather be unhappy in my love for you than never have seen you" (Alcoforado, 1893, Letter Three).

Hysteria

Hysteria is a neurotic response to the question of the difference between the sexes and to the enigma of the feminine sphere (Schaeffer, 2000). It only makes sense in the relation of the phallic position to the feminine sphere and the refusal to accept the feminine sphere. This is also the case when the hysteric is a man, but women are more sensitive and exposed to it.

It is an Oedipal neurosis par excellence due to its attempt to form a barrier against incest, because it conjures up the hated primal scene, and the interaction always involves three protagonists, with jealousy as the spice. The hysteric is in the position of the child as the excluded third party, who seeks to destroy any rapprochement between the couple, their own as well as that of others.

Hysterics are never where they are expected, so much so that their description and definition is elusive. One never knows what sex they claim to belong to, with the result that they have been attributed with bisexuality. It is understandable, on account of the predominance of this personality type in women, that hysteria has lent itself to certain pejorative descriptions of the feminine sphere. They practice "the art of running away" (Schaeffer, 2020).

Why the art? Hysteria, Freud said, is a "distorted work of art" (Freud, 1912-1913; Sollers, 1980). It has thus lent itself to all the fantasies of femininity idealized by men, those that have recognized themselves in the predominance of the auto-eroticism of thought and of imaginary life over real life. Baudelaire "cultivated his hysteria with excessive pleasure and terror," Sainte-Beuve spoke of his "moral hysteria," Flaubert described himself as a "big hysterical girl." During the fiftieth anniversary of hysteria, in 1928,

Aragon and Breton hailed it as "the greatest poetic discovery of the end of the 19th century."

If I have used the metaphor "rubies abhor red" (Schaeffer, 2018) for hysteria, it is because red is the colour that the ruby both rejects and exhibits, while absorbing all the other colours of the prism. It is to designate the type of defence employed by the hysterical ego violated by the libido, which consists in highlighting and exhibiting sexuality in order to defend itself against it. It is a flamboyant colour that also expresses the hysteric's attraction and seduction.

The hysterical woman remains fixed to the Oedipal conflict, to anxiety related to the difference between the sexes and to castration anxiety. Her excitement and passionate quest concern the enigma of the difference between the sexes, of the heterosexual relationship, and the secret of genital desire. The sense she has that something is eluding her, and her painful feeling of being excluded from it, gives rise in her to intolerable hatred of the primal scene.

This exacerbation of the Oedipal conflict thus keeps her fixed or regressed to the all-or-nothing opposition of the phallic monist phase, and thus to a primal scene between two protagonists, one of whom is phallic and the other castrated, and vice versa.

Through its theatrical aspects, provocations and permanent eroticization, hysteria abuses and empoisons itself,. and the whole circus is a struggle, a permanent defence against anxiety and depression. It is just as much "*belle indifférence*" as "*belle innocence,*" because it projects the conflict on to the other, who has the task of processing it.

Symptomatic hysteria is a symptomatology of the repudiated feminine sphere.

Eating disorders

The fact that the pathology of eating disorders – with their dual aspects of anorexia and bulimia – are predominant in adolescent girls (more than 95% are female), raises questions about the phenomena linked to feminine sexuality and its destiny of being open to large amounts of libidinal excitation (Schaeffer, 2002).

In girls, as I have already said, it is the belly, the inside of the body, that can be the object of anxiety, or threatened with destruction in fantasy, as theorized by Melanie Klein. It is threatened more by invasion and intrusion than by what can be torn away or cut off.

In eating disorder addictions, a confusion can be observed between drive and object, as well as a deterioration of the drive into excitation.

When the mother tends to confuse herself with the infant's oral impulses for too long, capturing them and so diverting their development, she does not allow the infant to experience its drive trajectory, to differentiate between drive and object, to effect the first internalizations of primary identification, or to differentiate between subject and object. The attachment is maintained at a fusional level. The mother is "unlosable," in the sense of the object-loss defined by Freud.

The mother/object cannot therefore be constituted by introjecting a representation, creating distance from the real object or by identification, but remains a persecuting incorporated object which cannot be assimilated, and whose self-destructive potential will be expressed by excesses in absorbing, expelling or refusing food, even to the point of defying death.

There is thus a search in the external non-human world for what was lacking in the first introjections of the maternal environment, for what was lacking in the first reciprocal seductions between mother and infant, which awaken and excite the reciprocal erogenous zones. This non-symmetrical tuning, when it exists, enables the erotic impulses both to draw support from the satisfaction of need and to disengage from it by becoming conflictualized.

In terms of incorporation, this lack of introjection will be expressed through the refusal, absorption or forced expulsion of an object that has been de-symbolized as a food product, and through the degradation of the drive into a need. The destructiveness inherent in this degradation manifests itself through a perversion of oral sexual impulses, and through defiance of the instincts of self-preservation, which can even result in letting oneself die.

The instinctual drive and the object are "faecalized" and fetishized as part-instincts, i.e. functioning independently, and as a part-objects. Like the fetish, the food object is inanimate, inhuman, always available, ready to be consumed or rejected at will; it can be destroyed in the process of consumption, and yet it is indestructible and renewable, like excrement.

We know the extent to which the relationship between anorexic and bulimic patients and their real mothers is one of passion, mutual control, love and destructive hatred, excluding the father. The absence of limits in relation to the mother imprisons the daughter in an incestuous relationship of mutual devouring and narcissistic seduction.

The part-object food serves to avoid both the anxiety of losing the primary object, by reducing it to the function of a wholly assimilable object, and the struggle against dependence on this primary object, by substituting dependence on a non-human object. The question is not one of the absence or presence of an envied penis, but rather of an empty or full interior, whose transition zones are not eroticized into erogenous zones. It is filling or emptying that is auto-eroticized.

In anorexia, everything is situated on the side of repression, whatever the cost. It is when it comes to cathecting sexual penetration and the erotic vagina that deficiencies in internalization and threats of a narcissistic breach may reappear. The predominantly female behavioural pathologies of anorexia and bulimia concern "anxieties related to the feminine sphere," to do with the opening and closing of the body, and testify to the failure to process them through introjection.

If the "large unfilled hole" (the expression of one of Binswanger's bulimic patients) cannot be constituted as an erogenous zone and a place of sexual penetration, it remains open to all winds, a place of anxiety and pregenital intrusion, where a narcissistic breach of the envelope of the boundaries of the ego occurs.

The bulimic responds by filling, the anorexic by closing all the exits and orifices. Getting pregnant early, in an adolescent, can also be a way of filling up and closing all the exits.

Depression

The depressive state (when we say we feel depressed, down or despondent) should be distinguished from its pathological form of depression (Schaeffer, 2013).There is less and less tolerance for the depressive state in today's society which pushes us towards an ideal of happiness and individual fulfilment, accentuating narcissism, the cult of the body and the ego ideal to the detriment of the superego as well as object and Oedipal relationships. Feelings of shame prevail over those of guilt. A lack of tolerance for depressive states can lead to overuse of antidepressants, which simply deprive people of the ability to use their own mental resources.

The depressive state leads us to talk about loss and the situation of dependence. We can see that the form of dependence, the meaning of loss, the loss of the object, the object of the loss, the object-related or narcissistic damage, and the expression of pain or suffering, often manifest themselves differently from one sex to another, and that this has an influence on the conditions of the onset of depression and the forms it takes.

It could be said that depression in a woman is linked to disappointed expectations, to the difficulty of symbolizing her sexual organs. When her primary erotogenic masochism is not well anchored, when it does not act as a safety-catch, the downfall can be profound and turn into melancholia. The disappointed expectation of a man's desire, the disappointed expectation of having a child, confronts her with feelings of emptiness: the emptiness of a body that is no longer inhabited by bodily narcissism, no longer illuminated by the gaze of a man's desire, or by the tenderness of a child.

Dependence, which can be concealed in presence, is revealed and suddenly discovered when lack becomes clearer, when confirmation by the object and its gaze disappears. In women, this reveals an object-loss confused with a total narcissistic loss. "If you leave me, I'll kill myself, I'll ruin myself… or else I'll remain alone." The solitude of women is a fact of society, whether it is chosen or suffered. Men rarely stay alone: the female object was first and foremost maternal… and it remains so.

Intrapsychic separations are narcissistic, object-related and erotic. They concern multiple objects: the self-image, phallic hyper-cathexis, dissociation of the feminine and maternal spheres, parental imagos, the illusion of omnipotence and immortality, etc. The psychical transformations they require can take the form of denial, narcissistic or relational overcompensation, depression, melancholia, etc., or libidinal reorganization.

A woman's total commitment to love, body and soul, which is just as common in some men, is very similar to that of the early days of life with the primary object. And the depressive state can hark back to the mourning that accompanies every experience of otherness. The other, is the one who emerges in hatred, the one who breaks the state of fusion; it can be the father, the baby brother or sister or … the Oedipal mother.

Why are we suddenly overcome by a feeling of sadness or despair, even though nothing serious has happened, nothing more than an allusion to a painful or overly happy past that evokes feelings of nostalgia? When, as the saying goes, "we have every reason to be happy," why do we suddenly feel that nothing is going right any more, that the joy of living has gone, that the meaning of life has been lost, that the motor of the libido has broken down, that belief in illusion is no longer possible, that the future is no longer of interest? It is impossible not to evoke a deferred effect of the primary relationship, the impossibility of mourning the maternal object.

Anxiety and depressive states are constitutive experiences of the human being, linked to internalization and human maturation, an attempt to master conflicts, disappointment or loss. Depressive feelings (the *grande tristezza* according to Dante) do not arise from a particular circumstance but from existence itself. It is due to the inevitable confrontation between human beings and life, to separations, uprootings, losses, to the feeling of our inadequacies, to the presence of evil, to the inevitability of death and ageing, to the experience of meaninglessness, to the experience of having reached one's limits. They serve as a "signal" marking an apparent insurmountable difficulty in confronting these trials.

The menopause

The onset of the menopause reactivates and exacerbates the question of the antagonism that exists in women between the erotic feminine sphere and the maternal sphere. Unlike the maternal sphere, which is periodic and temporal, the erotic feminine sphere is marked by the timelessness of the sexual drive, by its constant pressure. The maternal sphere is subject to a clock, while the feminine sphere is unending pressure.

Puberty and the menopause are the two limits of the biological period of procreation. It is a matter, therefore, of what marks female temporality, the rhythm and periodicity of the maternal feminine sphere.

Hélène Deutsch (1945) has compared the menopause to puberty, because it is a time for renouncing everything that was received during puberty. She observes overactivity, the resurgence of fantasies of rape and pregnancy, the need for emancipation, and equivalent symptoms, as if what is "too early" and what is "too late" coincided.

When the procreative organs cease to function, it may be experienced, during the crisis period, as a castration that has actually occurred. A woman then no longer feels capable of being either a mother or a woman, and she is not a man either.

If, at puberty, the onset of menstruation is experienced by some adolescent girls as a castration, this is a "red" castration, whereas that of the menopause is a "white" castration. It can take on "the colours of mourning, black or white: black as in depression, white as in states of emptiness" (Green, 2001, p. 174).

In fact, sensations of bodily transformation are accompanied, as in puberty, by feelings of uncanniness. The recognition of the body's image becomes blurred in the mirror. In both cases, it is a matter of mourning all possibilities, all illusions. During puberty, these include infantile megalomania and the fantasy of bisexuality, and during the menopause, the wish to rebuild one's life with a new man and new children. The sense of injustice in relation to men, for whom this is possible, reactivates envy, penis envy and castration anxiety.

This stage is the most difficult, because it requires a woman to undergo many psychical transformations which involve mourning childbirth, youth, the archaic mother and the Oedipal mother, children who have grown up, and parents who have died or are nearing the end of their lives.

The ordeal of the difference between the sexes irrupts again traumatically at this time of life, and needs to be worked through urgently: indeed, men and women are far from equal when it comes to the problems of procreation, erotic seduction and death.

Oedipal conflicts flare up again. The sense of injustice that women feel with regard to men, who have the possibility of rebuilding their lives with a young woman and children, reactivates the ordeal of the difference between the sexes, castration anxieties and the phallic solution of penis envy. Young women, who have all these possibilities ahead of them, can also experience these envious feelings. "The shadow that falls on the ego" is the shadow of a young and beautiful woman, which can give rise to hostile feelings in a mother towards her daughter. "Mirror, my beautiful mirror!" The object of rivalry is no longer the mother, but the daughter.

The "syndrome of the empty nest" is painful, especially for women who have not had children, but also for women for whom motherhood was the centre of their identity and who had projected all their phallic narcissism on their children. Separation anxiety begins well before, when the children begin to have their own love lives and confront their parents with a primal scene with its potential or excitation, abandonment and betrayal. When the children leave home, other losses, which were concealed by their presence, may then reemerge, such as the loss of a husband or the actual or potential loss of parents. A woman may begin to regret an abortion she had decades earlier. Refuge is often found in illness, physical suffering and somatization, with wounded narcissism taking its place and degrading or diverting the libido.

Depressive affects and psychic pain may be denied, often through acting out, hyperactivity or hysterical exacerbation.

For a certain number of women who extend or discover their erotic sex life with a man younger than themselves, according to Hélène Deutsch, this is a third revival of the Oedipal crisis, where the incestuous object becomes the son who is cathected with all the qualities of the ideal that she herself, as a little girl, had attributed to her own father.

The fifties are often marked by depression, either temporary or permanent, sometimes accompanied by anxiety, a hostile devaluation of one's own image and a loss of self-esteem. What was once possessed is lost, what was hoped for never happened.

"After women have lost their genital function," writes Freud (1913), "they become quarrelsome, vexatious, overbearing, petty and stingy; that is to say, they exhibit typically sadistic and anal-erotic traits which they did not possess earlier" (p. 323).

All traditional societies fear menopausal women. Françoise Héritier (1996) says that the menopausal woman is the person most likely to be accused of witchcraft. The fear of witches stems from the fact that they are not subject to a man who dominates them by giving them sexual satisfaction.

It is clear that this period is the most favourable time for cathexes involving sublimation of all kinds and grand-mothering activities, etc. However, how can one remain a woman when the sparkle of femininity declines and motherhood fades?

Could this not be a chance, an opportunity for women, freed from procreation and mothering, to free their bodies from that of their mothers, to mourn the loss of what their mother could not give them and what they unconsciously continue to expect from her, an expectation that they often prolong in relation to their partner, and with the analyst? The sacrifice offered to the archaic pregenital mother, as manifested by pathologies in the feminine sphere, such as anorexia/bulimia, and phenomena of frigidity or sterility, may no longer have any reason to exist. Could desire, which, due to the constant pressure of the drives, is indestructible, finally be permitted, and the eroticism of ecstatic pleasure be liberated? Could this mark the end of the maternal sphere, paving way for the feminine sphere at last? The question of the partner, however, remains.

If the menopause is a troublesome and censored subject, in my view it is because it harks back to the genitality of a woman, whose age allows her to picture the genitals and sexual ecstasy of her mother, which are taboo par excellence.

Neither a woman's social or erotic achievements can be achieved without conscious or unconscious guilt, without a sense of betrayal towards the family, perhaps in the same way as in adolescence. Perhaps we can say that the most important thing for a woman is to have been able, both physically and psychically, to have the three experiences of being a woman/subject, a mother and a lover, even if it means giving up the illusion of having them all with the same man?

References

Alcoforado, M. (1893). *The Letters of a Portuguese Nun*, trans. Edgar Prestage. London: David Nutt.

Deutsch, H. (1945). *The Psychology of Women, Vol 2, Motherhood*. New York, NY: Grune & Stratton.

Freud, S. (1912–1913). Totem and taboo. *S.E.* 13. London: Hogarth, pp. 1–161.

Freud, S. (1913). The disposition to obsessional neurosis. *S.E.* 12. London: Hogarth, pp. 317–326.

Green, A. (2001). The dead mother. In: *Life Narcissism, Death Narcissism*, trans. Andrew Weller. London: Free Association Books.

Héritier, F. (1996). *Masculin/féminin, la pensée de la différence*. Paris: Odile Jacob.

Labé, L. (2014). *Love Sonnets and Elegies*, trans. R. Sieburth. New York, NY: NYRB Poets.

Schaeffer, J. (2000). L'hystérie, une libido en crise face à la différence des sexes. *Revue française de psychosomatique*, 13: 107–138.

Schaeffer, J. (2002). Le féminin et l'alimentaire. In: *Perspectives Psy, Dossier: à propos de l'anorexie mentale: un débat franco-mexicain*, 41(1): 19–23. Paris: EDK.

Schaeffer, J. (2013). Le risque de la perte. Angoisses et dépression au féminin. In: *Monographies et Débats de Psychanalyse, La sexualité féminine*. Paris: Presses Universitaires de France, pp.109–128.

Schaeffer, J. (2018/2011). *The Universal Refusal: A Psychoanalytic Exploration of the Feminine Sphere and Its Repudiation*, trans. D. Alcorn. London: Routledge.

Schaeffer, J. (2020). L'art de la fugue. Preface to Benyamin, M. (2020). *L'hystérie, Entre séduction et dépression*. Paris: In Press.

Sollers, P. (1980). L'hystérique a toujours raison. Preface to the Italian edition of Charcot, J-M., & Richer, P. (1887). *Les démoniaques dans l'art*. Paris: Delahaye et Lecrosnier.

Chapter 9

Feminine derailments

The risks

Among the possible feminine derailments, I have chosen to deal only with passion in love and feminine perversion. Many themes are therefore left aside. Some of them are dealt with in this book, such as envy and jealousy, the problem of incest, hate and destructiveness. I will look at the taboos in the feminine sphere, and insist on the inescapable transgression represented by the feminine sphere itself.

Passion in love

Suddenly, it is love at first sight. A sudden desire wells up. A choice has to be made. All this escapes us. Suddenly, something one had always known but never formulated comes flooding back with force and clarity. A crazy idea comes to mind: "*This is the man or woman of my life.*" Then, the I no longer exists, there's just me and him or her.

Passion is based on a sense of lack, of incompleteness (Schaeffer, 2018a, 2018b). Everyone loves in order to be loved. But passion is always asymmetrical. The passionate person loves to love, but more secretly, he also loves not to love and not to be loved. What matters most is the sway he has over his object. While love can become knowledge, passion remains ignorance or misrecognition.

The nature of falling head over heels in love that forms the basis of this sudden madness is deeply rooted in our earliest experiences and perceptions, in the archaic infantile attachment. When people are madly in love, both of them experience the erasure of their own boundaries, as in early childhood when the infant does not yet know that it exists outside its mother. The other becomes the reason for living, the cause of every happiness and every torment.

We all know what the first passionate, unconditional experience of love is, the one that only makes sense when it is lost and triggers eternal longings for reunion. It is the first love sickness.

Passionate love is a "transference" which, in analysis, will be expressed with all the misrecognition of the subject and of the other to whom the demand for love is addressed. It can become a passionate, erotomanic, mad transference.

DOI: 10.4324/9781003471042-9

The other, at first a contingent object of desire, becomes for the person who is passionately in love an essential, all-powerful object of need, an "absolute master" who merges with the representation of death, since he or she is absolutely dependent on this other.

In the words of the poet, Alphonse de Lamartine [1790–1869], *"When you're missing just one person, the whole world feels empty!"* In fact, this person who you are missing is first and foremost yourself. It is the absolute fear of being abandoned that guides the emotional life of these subjects, even if they try to protect themselves against it.

The experience of passion is to some extent independent of the qualities of the object, or even of its presence. The person in the throes of passion cathects another person, or their image, as the embodiment of their ideal; they love only their own creation, their idealized double. By placing a person at the centre of their life, they enjoy this greatness vicariously and through identification. This allows them to ignore the aspects of the other in themselves by returning to the illusion of a person undivided by their psychic conflictuality, and to experience intensely the illusion of psychic reunification, and its ecstatic pleasure.

If there is violence, if the suffering is unbearable, it is because we have projected the best of ourselves onto the other person. Any break-up is therefore experienced as a tear in our being, or worse, as a death wish on the part of the other person. The risk of melancholia is real.

There is a passion for passion, a love for the suffering that the other always inflicts on you, precisely because he or she is "other." Hence this illogical and painful trap: the other becomes the only remedy for the evil of which he or she is the cause.

All passion contains a core of destruction and death; indeed, the death drive is at work in the experience of "losing oneself with the other." It is here that it makes itself heard the most, through two aspects: ascendancy over the other, and self-sacrifice and self-destruction.

Jealousy gives us the right to kill, even to kill ourselves in order to stop suffering from this lack. In some cases, separation is impossible because the passionate tie protects the subject against the death drive and its derivative, annihilation.

A female perversion?

The male pervert is described as someone who claims to control simultaneously the phallus, the castration anxiety aroused by the difference between the sexes, and the primal scene.

Can one speak of a specifically feminine perversion? (Schaeffer, 2003) What would a woman claim to control since, according to Freud, she has no castration anxiety because she has nothing to lose at the level of her genitals, but rather a castration complex in the form of penis envy. This envy can lead her to control a man's penis, to castrate him. But what is it that has to be controlled?

A man struggles against his castration anxiety by means of a part-object that has phallic significance and stands in for the phallus, something that is extra and external, that is intended to represent castration and the absence of castration. It could be a boot, braid chopping, a car, or a woman to show off. Does a woman struggle against her anxiety related to the feminine sphere, to penetration, to being opened up by means of a part-object that refers to the interior, to the hollow space, to the inside?

First form of feminine perversion

It concerns what the woman is penetrated by, what she can or cannot control: the penis, the child, food, etc.

- Maternal perversion can be exercised on the real object that is the child. Even if we consider as Freud does, that this child is a substitute in fantasy for the penis, I believe that it refers to another more specifically feminine dimension, namely, what is interior, inside the body, just as the female sexual organs are inside the body, and as the infant was during pregnancy, but also inside in the sense of movements of penetration and devouring. All this brings into play the psychical processes of incorporation, introjection and internalization.
- Appetite perversion is the one that best illustrates what, in the relationship to the fetishistic object, to the part-object, is specific to the difference between the sexes. The advantage of food is that it can be given at will and is easily controlled. Like the fetish, the food object is inanimate, inhuman, always available, ready to be consumed or rejected at will; it can be destroyed in the process of consumption and yet it is indestructible, renewable, like faeces.

Second form of feminine perversion

This perversion exacerbates and deflects the specificity of feminine sexuality, and its capacity to introject large quantities of libidinal energy. It concerns a perversion with erotomanic tendencies, perverse masochism and moral masochism.

- Perversion with erotomanic tendencies refers to a female tendency towards passion for love, a love of love and idealization of the object. This tendency is due to the formation of the female Oedipus complex, which requires a change of object and a violent uprooting from the pregenital relationship with the mother. Perversions with erotomanic tendencies include "Don Juans," nymphomaniacs and women who are said to be "crazy about their bodies."

- Masochistic perversion. If masochism plays a role in the most feminine form of sexual perversion, it is because it nestles at the heart of a woman's ecstatic pleasure. If women are often chosen to serve as sadistic partners for masochistic men, it is undoubtedly because they represent the all-powerful anal and phallic mother, but also because they know a lot about what masochism is, and it is masochism that leads the way.
- Moral masochism can also figure among female perversions, when it manifests repeated and passionate enjoyment in being mistreated.

The key to male perversion is the veneration of the phallus; the key to female perversion is the veneration/hatred of the archaic mother. And, as has been clinically observed, perversion appears to be a defence, a bulwark, perhaps more fragile in women than in men, against the dangers of depressive and psychotic narcissistic breakdown.

Taboos of the feminine sphere

"It could almost be said that woman as a whole is taboo...." In what sense is the feminine sphere marked by this sacred, consecrated, impure and therefore dangerous character as soon as the rites of avoidance and prohibition are transgressed (Schaeffer, 2006)?

In his article "The taboo of virginity," Freud (1918) distinguishes three elements. The first is the taboo of blood, particularly that of women: the blood of deflowering, menstruation, childbirth, etc. The second is stranger-anxiety, anxiety related to everything that is new, unexpected and disturbing, like the first act of sexual intercourse. The third taboo embraces sexual life as a whole.

I have insisted, in particular, on the taboo of "seeing." "There is one technique," writes Freud (1933), "which women may have invented, that of plaiting and weaving... Nature itself would seem to have given the model which this achievement imitates by causing the growth at maturity of the pubic hair that conceals the genitals" (p. 132).

The special interest Freud accorded to the visual is well known: his interest for visual representation, dream images, the role of hallucinatory functioning, the scopic instinct, curiosity, the passion for seeing and knowing, and so on.

Freud defines curiosity, the urge for knowledge, as an extension of the child's interest in his own sexual organs and those of his parents, of his quest concerning the enigma of the difference between the sexes. The mother's sexual organ is at the heart of the enigma. "Mummy, have you got a widdler?" asks Hans, "Of course, why?" she replies. The child spies on everything that goes in and out of his mother's sexual organ. When he later sees a bloodstained bedpan after his little sister's delivery, he says: "But blood doesn't come out of my widdler." This is the boy's castration anxiety when faced with women's blood.

Pilosity is also a subject of taboo; that is to say, the object that is supposed to conceal, rather than the one that must be concealed. Is it a return of the repressing force in place of the repressed? I would say it is more a question of suppression. The hair that marked the onset of puberty, of the emergence of genital sexuality, takes on the heritage of the obscenity of the female genitals. What is sexual bait, what must remain hidden, is displaced on to pilosity and hair.

A Muslim patient, who presented with a vaginal symptom, said: "When I had my hair cut, I had the impression that I no longer had any genitals." The veil of fundamentalist Muslims must cover all of a woman's hair; there must be no manifest sign of female temptation. Their pubic hair is carefully plucked, shaved. In some Jewish Chassidic communities, married women have their heads shaven and wear a wig. The inquisitors who hunted witches in the Middle Ages shaved hysterical women, who were believed to be hiding the fornicating Devil in their pubic hair.

The blood taboo covers almost the whole of a woman's life. It presides over the destiny of both her feminine and maternal spheres. It is the "red thread of women's blood" (Schaeffer, 2005). This cyclical blood rises and falls like the faces of the moon, fluctuating like the tides, seasons and harvests. It is called the "climacteric." Hence the taboo, and the sacred characteristic attached to it; some people attribute a similar characteristic to climatic phenomena whose generosity is fertile and invoked, such as the sun or the rain, but also to events whose dangerousness is feared, such as cyclones, tidal waves and tsunamis. These cataclysms are often given women's names: Katrina, Rita, and so on.

The blood of menstruation condenses all the dangers and all the taboos. It brings together sexuality, procreation and death, thus the Oedipal prohibitions and cultural prohibitions against incest and patricide. It covers the anxieties related to the feminine sphere as well as those of castration and death. This blood can only be impure and evil. The blood of menstruation is incoagulable, which leads to death. There is a parallel between the rituals surrounding menstruation and death.

The menstruating woman thus destroys everything that she is supposed to protect and produce as mother earth. In short, she destroys life just as she destroys the child that she is not bearing. Behind the taboo of blood is hidden, therefore, the fear inspired by the dark forces of life and death, those of an omnipotent, suffocating and devouring archaic mother who has the exclusive right to give life and take it back again.

Men then created myths and rituals designed to exorcise and control the malevolence of women: social rites of isolation, medical rites of expulsion, religious rites of purification. *Inter urinas et faeces nascimur* [We are born between urine and faeces] declared the Church Fathers, where the locus of procreation and the locus of ejection merge.

It is therefore an area of confusion, hence the fascination and fear it can inspire due to the danger of dissolving into formlessness, and to the hidden sources that emerge inside the woman's body. Menstruation is taboo in almost all civilizations. The taboo conveys the ambivalence between the impure and the sacred. It combines voluptuousness and the fear of touching.

A woman is both sacred and impure: sacred when she is a virgin; a mother, a Madonna, impure when she is a woman, throughout her sexual life, from her first menstruation to the menopause. Herein lies the split between the mother and whore. She is therefore doubly taboo, doubly untouchable.

The feminine sphere as a transgression of laws and taboos

How could the emancipation of women be brought about other than through the transgression of laws and taboos?

Nothing makes sense if we neglect to take into account the prohibitions and taboos that affect women's bodies, their sexuality, and their role in marriage and motherhood. Numerous prohibitions and taboos still dominate women's bodies, their sexuality and their role in marriage and motherhood. Certain rites govern their blood. Prohibitions against contraception and abortion remain a threat; they were forbidden in France up until 1975.

In other parts of the world, women are subjected to numerous sexual prohibitions; they are forced to undergo excision, infibulation and stoning. Only sterile and menopausal women acquire a degree of public authority, while men reclaim the power to procreate and control children.

Religious taboos in the three monotheistic religions still subject women to rites of purity and impurity: they are forbidden access to religious services, their sexuality is forbidden outside marriage and restricted to procreation, polygamy and repudiation still exist, divorce is forbidden, and so on. Not to mention the persecution inflicted by the inquisitors in the past, particularly in Spain. Outside these monotheistic religions, only Tantric Buddhism in Tibet accords status to a women's ecstatic pleasure.

But women's main conquest has been to be able to consciously separate their erotic desire from their desire to procreate, and to be able to decide for themselves whether or not to have children.

Women's ecstatic pleasure can only be transgressive, subversive and beyond the limits because it does not obey the phallic law, because it is another form of *jouissance* (*une jouissance "Autre"*) according to Jacques Lacan.

How could the erotic feminine sphere fail to be transgressive?

A daughter's first transgression is her betrayal of the primitive, omnipotent mother, that of the primal homosexual relationship. It means turning away from her to expect from the father what she is not or no longer capable of giving him. What is involved is a castration of the phallic maternal imago.

Lacan speaks of the mother/daughter "ravage." The love/hate attachment reflects the daughter's difficulty of freeing herself from the maternal hold. Separating herself from a primary maternal object, due to the necessity for both identification and deidentification, carries the risk of losing a part of herself.

The second transgression is directed at the Oedipal mother, out of rivalry concerning the desire to seduce the father, and the expectation in fantasy of receiving from him the promise of a child, or the promise of ecstatic pleasure.

A little girl can make early use of her femininity and her power of seduction, seducing not only her father but also her mother, in an inverted Oedipus situation. In this way, she can satisfy her need for recognition of her feminine being and as a sexual being in her own right.

References

Freud, S. (1918 [1917]). The taboo of virginity (contributions to the psychology of love, III). *S. E. 11*. London: Hogarth, pp. 193–208.

Freud, S. (1933 [1932]). New introductory lectures on psychoanalysis. *S.E.* 22. London: Hogarth, pp. 7–182.

Schaeffer, J. (2003). Une perversion au féminin? *Groupal, 12*: 113–133. Paris: Publication du Collège de Psychanalyse Groupale et Familiale.

Schaeffer, J. (2005). Le fil rouge du sang de la femme. *Champ psychosomatique* 40: 39–64.

Schaeffer, J. (2006). Le tabou du féminin. In: *Monographies et Débats de Psychanalyse, Interdit et Tabou.* Paris: Presses Universitaires de France, pp. 171–199.

Schaeffer, J. (2018a). Passion amoureuse, folie ordinaire ou extraordinaire? In: Pommier, F. (Ed.) *La folie ordinaire.* Paris: Compagne Première, pp. 95–103.

Schaeffer, J. (2018b). Amour, passion et emprise sexuelle. In: Chaboudez, G., & Sédat, J. (Eds.) *Figures de la psychanalyse, Penser le sexuel (II)*. Paris: Érès, pp. 13–24.

Chapter 10

The otherness of the feminine sphere

What can be said about an encounter between the two sexes? At stake is the otherness of the feminine sphere, which the subject must tame in himself and in the other, whether he is a man or a woman. Otherwise, how can we avoid sliding towards devaluation, contempt, fear or hatred of the feminine sphere, to the point of their potential for destructive violence? And how can men and women not be drawn towards the familiar divide between mother and whore, or, why not… towards homosexuality?

Unlike the phallic/masculine pairing which, just like the anal/faecal pairing, supports the maintenance of social organization and its relations of power and domination, the constitution of a masculine/feminine pairing is a psychic creation, which implies the recognition and confrontation of otherness in the difference between the sexes. The ability to transform a phallic/castrated pairing into a masculine/feminine pairing determines the mode and quality of the sexual, affective and social relationship that is established between a man and a woman, and bears witness to a "work of culture."

How can we understand that this "repudiation of the feminine sphere," which Freud diagnosed in the twilight of his life, is still so widespread and persistent today? Why do women represent such a danger for social organization that it was necessary for a long time to exclude them from the public domain and to assume control over their erotic capacities and their procreative capacities? And why was everything related to power and knowledge considered for so long to be the preserve of men? One of the dangers is said to be that equality could induce confusion between the sexes and therefore destabilize sexual relations, and consequently the domination of one sex over the other.

Can we infer that what has always threatened the political, social and religious order concerns women's power to procreate, and even more so their erotic capacities? And, further, that what is intolerable is the representation of a mother/woman and woman/mother interpenetration. We know, incidentally, the extent to which the maternal sphere can seek, in both sexes, to countercathect the erotic feminine sphere!

The status of women is the mirror of the structure and history of a civilization, the pivot and revealer of what is changing in a society, the symptom of

DOI: 10.4324/9781003471042-10

crises and power struggles between the sexes, the emblem of all equality. Just as the fight for equality between the sexes is imperative and must be waged constantly in the social, political and economic spheres, so it can be harmful and damaging in the sexual sphere if it tends to merge with the abolition of the difference between the sexes, which must be exalted on account of the antagonism between the libido and the defences of the ego.

The phallic position concerns both sexes. Equating the phallic position with the masculine sphere is a necessity for the boy's first cathexis of his penis, but when it comes to the adult sexual encounter, phallic and masculine become antagonists. The feminine sphere is not opposed to the masculine sphere but to the phallic position.

My reflections on the feminine and the maternal spheres lead me to propose a metapsychological definition of the feminine sphere.

This "work of the feminine sphere" puts to the test the capacity of the ego in both sexes to admit and allow itself to be penetrated by large quantities of unbound excitation, without incurring a traumatic breach. The ego is thereby nourished and required to develop, enrich itself and grow. This is what I have called "non-dangerous de-liaisons."

This feminine capacity supports ecstatic pleasure, but also the high-energy bodily experiences of the maternal dimension of women, such as pregnancy and childbirth, as well as their experiences of mental life. This capacity for endurance certainly has an effect on the favourable growth of a child, and is probably one of the reasons why women live longer than men.

The other sex, whether one is a man or a woman, is always the feminine sex. Beyond the phallic position, then, is the feminine sphere.

Index